GAPS COOKBOOK FOR GUT HEALTH

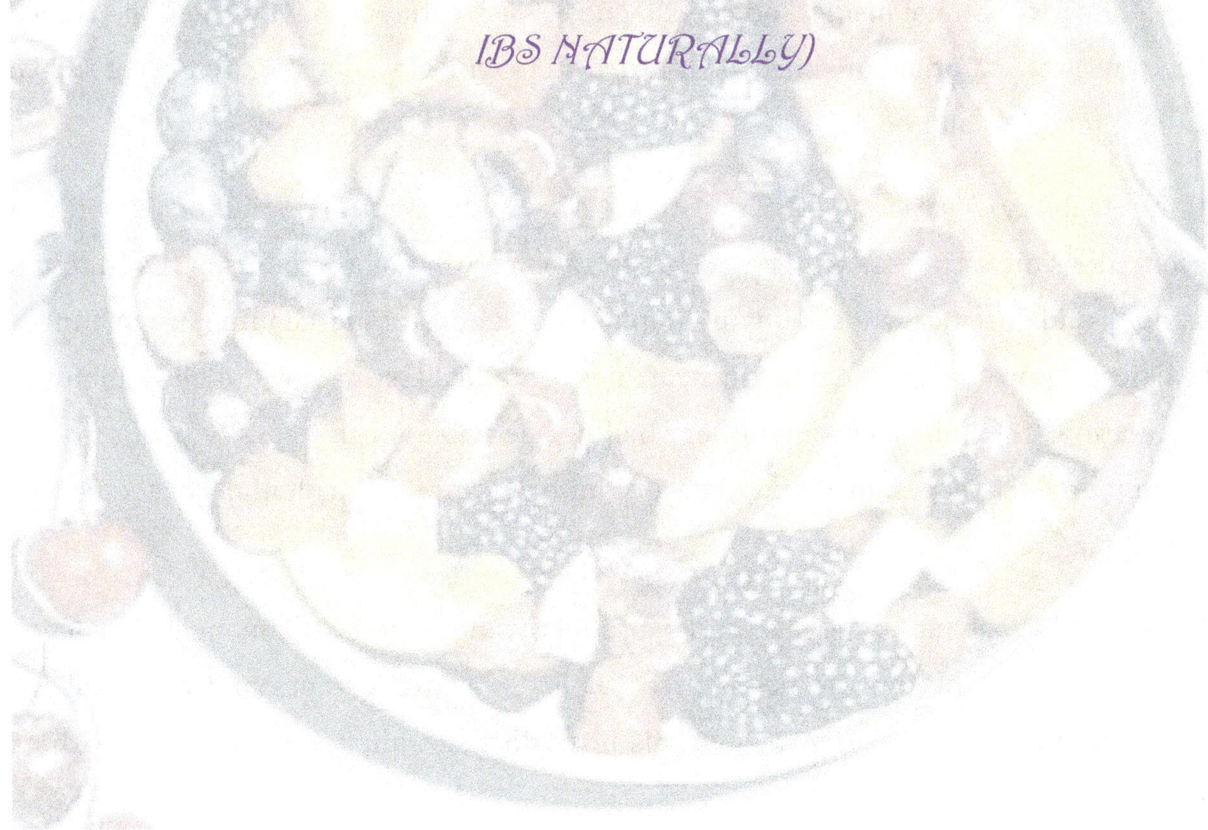

UNLOCK DIGESTIVE FREEDOM & RELIEVE AUTOIMMUNE SYMPTOMS, PLANT-BASED GAPS DIET RECIPES FOR HEALING & GUT HEALTH (GLUTEN & GRAIN-FREE, LOW-FODMAP, TREAT IBS NATURALLY)

Copyright © 2024 by DR Jane T. Ryan

INTRODUCTION TO GAPS DIET

The GAPS (Gut and Psychology Syndrome) Diet is a nutritional protocol designed to support gut health and address various physical and mental health conditions. Developed by Dr. Natasha Campbell-McBride, it emphasizes the connection between the gut and overall well-being.

Key Principles:

- Gut-Brain Connection: GAPS Diet recognizes the intricate link between the gut and the brain, suggesting that a compromised gut can contribute to various neurological and psychological disorders.

- Healing the Gut: The diet focuses on healing the gut lining by removing inflammatory foods and introducing nutrient-dense, easy-to-digest foods.

- Elimination of Certain Foods: GAPS advocates the removal of processed foods, sugar, grains, and other potential irritants to reduce inflammation and promote gut healing.

- Introduction of Nutrient-Rich Foods: The diet encourages the consumption of probiotic-rich foods, bone broth, fermented vegetables, and other nutrient-dense options to support a healthy gut microbiome.

Conditions Addressed by GAPS:

- Digestive Disorders: GAPS Diet is commonly recommended for individuals with digestive issues such as leaky gut syndrome, irritable bowel syndrome (IBS), and inflammatory bowel diseases (IBD).

- Behavioral and Neurological Disorders: Dr. Campbell-McBride suggests that the diet may have positive effects on conditions like autism, ADHD, and other behavioral and neurological disorders.

- Autoimmune Conditions: Some proponents believe that GAPS Diet can help manage autoimmune conditions by reducing inflammation and supporting immune function.

Implementation:

- Stages of GAPS Diet: The protocol is typically divided into stages, starting with an introductory phase that focuses on easily digestible foods and gradually introducing more complex foods as the gut heals.

- Supplementation: Alongside dietary changes, GAPS may include supplementation with probiotics, fish oil, and other nutrients to support gut health and overall well-being.

The GAPS Diet offers a holistic approach to health by recognizing the vital role of the gut in various bodily functions. While it has gained popularity for its potential benefits, it's crucial to consult with a healthcare professional before starting the diet, especially for individuals with pre-existing health conditions.

UNDERSTANDING GUT HEALTH

Understanding gut health is crucial for overall well-being. The gut, or gastrointestinal tract, is a complex system comprising the stomach, small intestine, and large intestine. It is essential for immune system function, nutrition absorption, and digestion.

Microbiome Composition:

- Trillions of bacteria, referred to as the microbiome, reside in the gut These include bacteria, viruses, fungi, and other microbes. The balance and diversity of these microorganisms are essential for maintaining a healthy gut.

Impact on Digestion:

- A healthy gut facilitates effective digestion. Enzymes and bacteria in the digestive tract break down food, allowing the body to absorb essential nutrients. Imbalances in the microbiome can lead to digestive issues such as bloating, gas, and constipation.

Immune System Connection:

- The gut plays a crucial role in supporting the immune system. A well-balanced microbiome helps prevent the overgrowth of harmful bacteria and supports the development of a robust immune response. Imbalances in the gut microbiome may contribute to autoimmune diseases and allergies.

Influence on Mental Health:

- The gut and the brain communicate with each other in both directions through the gut-brain connection Emerging research suggests that imbalances in the gut microbiome may influence mental health conditions such as anxiety and depression. The gut produces neurotransmitters that impact mood and cognitive function.

Dietary Impact on Gut Health:

- The gut microbiome is significantly impacted by diet. Consuming a diverse range of fiber-rich foods, fruits, vegetables, and fermented foods supports the growth of beneficial bacteria. On the contrary, diets high in processed foods and low in fiber can lead to an imbalance in the microbiome.

Probiotics and Prebiotics:

- Consuming sufficient amounts of live bacteria can yield health advantages, known as probiotics. Fermented foods such as sauerkraut, kefir, and yogurt contain them. Prebiotics, on the other hand, are non-digestible fibers that promote the growth of beneficial bacteria.

Factors Affecting Gut Health:

- Various factors can impact gut health, including antibiotics, stress, lack of sleep, and certain medications. Antibiotics, while necessary in some cases, can disrupt the balance of the microbiome by killing both harmful and beneficial bacteria.

Maintaining Gut Health:

- Adopting a gut-friendly lifestyle involves a combination of factors. This includes a balanced diet, regular exercise, stress management, and adequate sleep. Incorporating fermented foods and considering probiotic supplements can also support gut health.

Understanding gut health involves recognizing the intricate relationship between the microbiome, digestion, immune function, mental health, and overall well-being. By making informed lifestyle choices and prioritizing a gut-friendly diet, individuals can promote a healthy and balanced gut microbiome.

BASICS OF THE GAPS PROTOCOL

The GAPS (Gut and Psychology Syndrome) Protocol is a nutritional program designed to address gut health issues and their potential impact on mental and physical well-being. Developed by Dr. Natasha Campbell-McBride, a neurologist and nutritionist, the GAPS

Protocol focuses on healing the gut to improve overall health. Here are the basics of the GAPS Protocol:

Understanding GAPS:

- The GAPS Protocol is based on the concept that many health conditions, including neurological and psychological disorders, have their roots in an imbalanced and compromised gut. GAPS encompasses a range of conditions, from digestive disorders to neurological issues such as autism, ADHD, and depression.

Leaky Gut Syndrome:

- A central concept in the GAPS Protocol is "Leaky Gut Syndrome," where the intestinal lining becomes permeable, allowing toxins and undigested particles to enter the bloodstream. This is believed to trigger immune responses and inflammation, contributing to various health problems.

Importance of Gut Flora:

- The protocol emphasizes the significance of a healthy balance of gut flora. A diverse and well-balanced microbiome is crucial for proper digestion, nutrient absorption, and supporting the immune system. Imbalances in gut bacteria are thought to contribute to the development of GAPS-related conditions.

Introduction Diet:

- The GAPS Protocol typically starts with an Introduction Diet, which consists of easily digestible foods like homemade broths, fermented foods, and cooked vegetables. This phase aims to soothe and heal the gut lining while providing essential nutrients.

GAPS Diet Stages:

- The GAPS Diet progresses through several stages, gradually reintroducing more complex foods as the gut heals. It includes nutrient-dense foods like bone broth, probiotic-rich fermented foods, organic meats, and certain vegetables. The protocol advises avoiding processed foods, grains, and sugars.

Bone Broth and Fermented Foods:

- Bone broth is a cornerstone of the GAPS Protocol due to its rich nutrient content, including collagen and amino acids that support gut healing. Fermented foods like sauerkraut, kimchi, and yogurt introduce beneficial probiotics to aid in restoring a healthy microbiome.

Supplements:

- The protocol often recommends specific supplements to support gut healing and address nutritional deficiencies. This may include probiotics, fish oil, digestive enzymes, and vitamins and minerals that play a role in overall health.

Lifestyle Considerations:

- Beyond dietary changes, the GAPS Protocol emphasizes lifestyle factors such as stress management, quality sleep, and avoiding environmental toxins. These elements are considered essential for comprehensive healing and maintaining long-term health.

Individualized Approach:

- The GAPS Protocol acknowledges that each person is unique, and the approach may need to be adapted based on individual health issues, sensitivities, and responses. Working with healthcare professionals familiar with the protocol is often recommended.

Gradual Healing Process:

- Healing with the GAPS Protocol is seen as a gradual process. Depending on the severity of gut issues and associated health conditions, individuals may need to follow the protocol for an extended period. Regular monitoring and adjustments are made based on progress.

The GAPS Protocol is a comprehensive and individualized approach to healing the gut and addressing a range of health issues. While it has gained popularity, it's important for individuals to consult with healthcare professionals before starting the protocol to ensure it aligns with their specific health needs and conditions.

1
Broths and Stocks

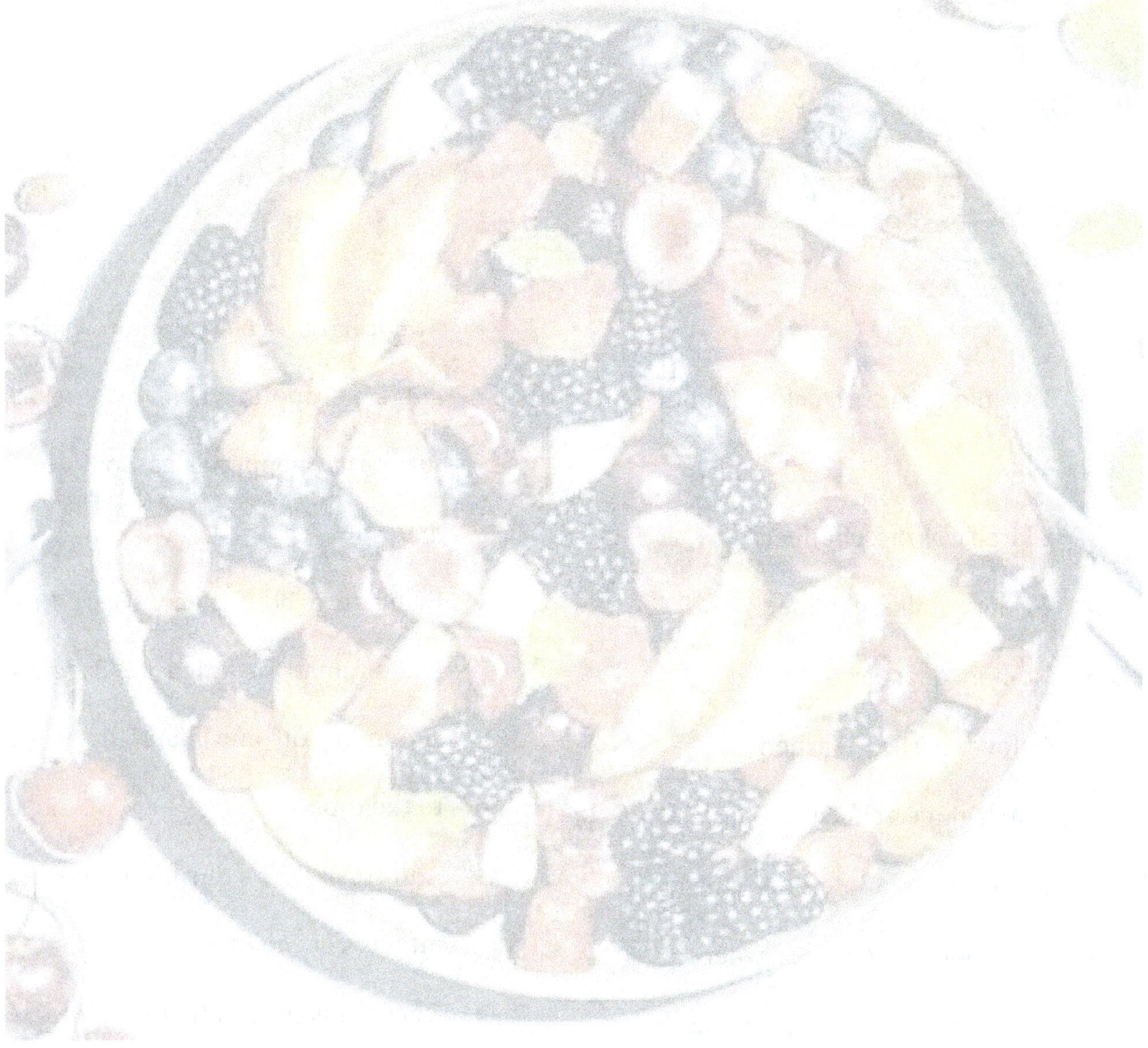

Healing Chicken Broth

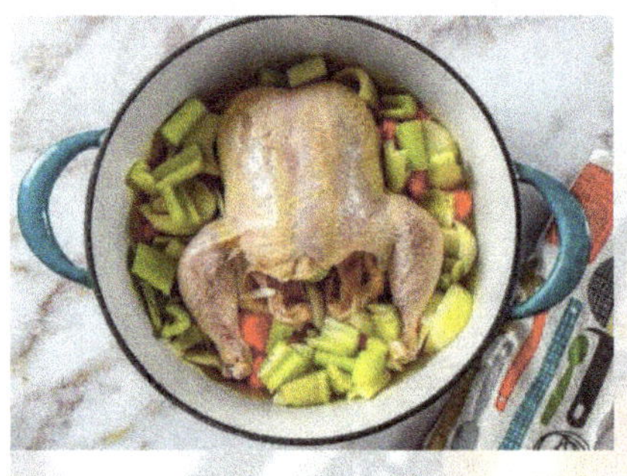

Ingredients:

- 1 whole organic chicken (about 3-4 lbs)
- 2 large carrots, chopped
- 2 celery stalks, chopped
- 1 onion, quartered
- 4 cloves garlic, smashed
- 1 inch ginger, sliced
- 1 tablespoon apple cider vinegar
- 1 teaspoon turmeric powder
- 1 teaspoon black peppercorns
- 1 bay leaf
- Fresh herbs (parsley, thyme, rosemary)
- Salt to taste

Procedure:

- Put the chicken in a big pot and add water to cover it.
- Add carrots, celery, onion, garlic, ginger, apple cider vinegar, turmeric, peppercorns, bay leaf, and salt.
- Bring to a boil, then reduce heat and simmer for at least 2-3 hours, skimming off any foam that rises to the top.
- Add fresh herbs during the last 30 minutes of cooking.
- Once cooked, strain the broth to remove solids, leaving a clear liquid.

Time of Preparation:

- Approximately 3-4 hours

Tips and Tricks:

- Use organic, free-range chicken for richer flavor and more nutrients.
- To aid in the removal of minerals from the bones, mix in a small amount of apple cider vinegar.
- Experiment with additional herbs and spices for personalized taste.

Nutritional Value (per serving):

- Calories: Approximately 60-80 kcal
- Protein: 8-10g
- Healthy Fats: 2-4g
- Carbohydrates: 4-6g

Health Benefits:

- Boosts immune system
- Supports gut health
- Rich in collagen for joint health
- Anti-inflammatory properties

Packaging and Storing:

- Allow the broth to cool before storing in airtight containers.
- Refrigerate for up to 4-5 days or freeze for longer shelf life.
- Consider freezing in ice cube trays for convenient portioning.

Precautions:

- Avoid excessive salt; adjust to taste gradually.
- Ensure the chicken is thoroughly cooked.
- If allergic to any ingredient, omit or replace accordingly.

Post Caution:

- Reheat the broth gently to preserve nutrients.

- Consume within a week for optimal freshness.

- Fresh herbs (thyme, rosemary, parsley)

- Salt to taste

Nutrient-Rich Beef Stock

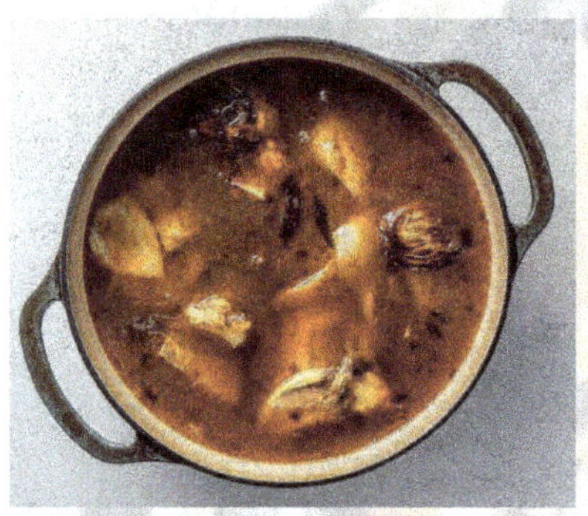

Ingredients:

- 2-3 lbs beef bones (marrow and knuckle bones)

- 2 carrots, chopped

- 2 celery stalks, chopped

- 1 onion, quartered

- 4 cloves garlic, smashed

- 1 tablespoon apple cider vinegar

- 1 teaspoon black peppercorns

- 2 bay leaves

Procedure:

- Roast beef bones in the oven at 400°F (200°C) for 30-40 minutes until browned.

- Place bones in a large pot, add vegetables, garlic, apple cider vinegar, peppercorns, bay leaves, and salt.

- Cover with water, bring to a boil, then simmer for at least 4-6 hours, skimming off any impurities.

- Add fresh herbs during the last hour of cooking.

- Strain the stock to remove solids, leaving a clear, rich liquid.

Time of Preparation:

- Approximately 4-6 hours

Tips and Tricks:

- Use bones with marrow for added richness and nutrients.
- Roasting bones enhances flavor.
- Add a splash of apple cider vinegar for mineral extraction.

Nutritional Value (per serving):

- Calories: Approximately 40-60 kcal
- Protein: 5-8g
- Healthy Fats: 2-4g
- Collagen: 1-2g

Health Benefits:

- Supports bone and joint health
- Provides essential minerals
- Boosts collagen intake for skin and gut health

Packaging and Storing:

- Allow the stock to cool before storing in airtight containers.
- Refrigerate for up to 5 days or freeze for long-term storage.
- Freeze in various portion sizes for flexibility.

Precautions:

- Monitor salt content to avoid excess sodium.
- Ensure bones are from a reliable, grass-fed source.
- Filter out impurities during the cooking process.

Post Caution:

- Reheat gently to preserve nutrients.
- Consume within a week for optimal freshness.

Vegetable Broth for Gut Support

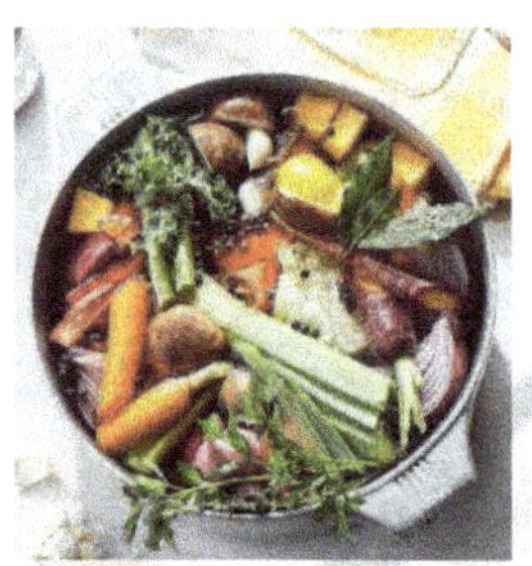

Ingredients:

- 2 large carrots, chopped
- 2 celery stalks, chopped
- 1 large leek, sliced
- 1 zucchini, sliced
- 1 cup spinach or kale, chopped
- 1 tomato, quartered
- 4 cloves garlic, minced
- 1-inch ginger, grated
- 1 tablespoon olive oil
- 1 tablespoon apple cider vinegar
- 1 teaspoon turmeric powder
- 1 teaspoon cumin seeds
- 1 bay leaf
- Fresh herbs (parsley, cilantro, dill)
- Salt to taste

Procedure:

- In a large pot, heat olive oil and sauté garlic, ginger, and leek until fragrant.
- Add carrots, celery, zucchini, tomato, and continue sautéing for 5-7 minutes.
- Pour in enough water to cover the vegetables, add apple cider vinegar, turmeric, cumin seeds, bay leaf, and salt.
- Bring to a boil, then reduce heat and simmer for 1-2 hours, allowing flavors to meld.
- Add fresh herbs during the last 15 minutes of cooking.
- Strain the broth, retaining the liquid while discarding solids.

Time of Preparation:

- Approximately 1-2 hours

Tips and Tricks:

- Use organic vegetables for a cleaner broth.
- Experiment with different herbs for diverse flavors.
- Include gut-friendly spices like ginger and turmeric.

Nutritional Value (per serving):

- Calories: Approximately 20-30 kcal
- Fiber: 2-4g
- Vitamins A, C, K: Abundant
- Antioxidants: High

Health Benefits:

- Supports gut health and digestion
- Provides a range of vitamins and minerals
- Anti-inflammatory properties

Packaging and Storing:

- Cool the broth before storing in airtight containers.
- Refrigerate for up to 4-5 days or freeze for extended shelf life.
- Freeze in smaller portions for convenience.

Precautions:

- Adjust salt levels carefully to avoid excessive sodium intake.
- Ensure all vegetables are thoroughly washed.
- Tailor the recipe to accommodate individual dietary restrictions.

Post Caution:

- Reheat gently to retain nutrients.
- Consume within a week for optimal freshness

2

Fermented Foods

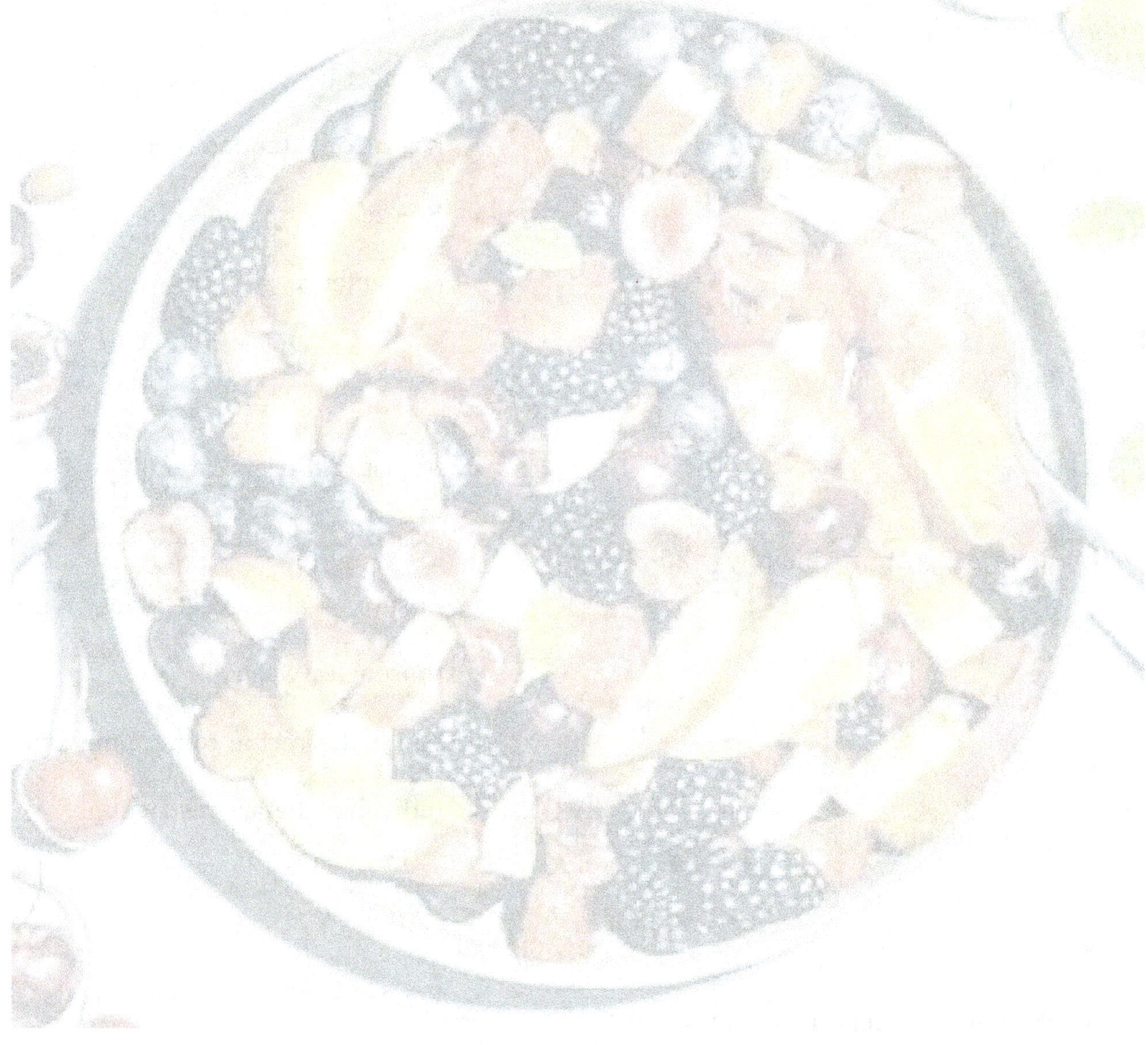

20 | GAPS COOKBOOK FOR GUT HEALTH

Sauerkraut with Probiotic Goodness

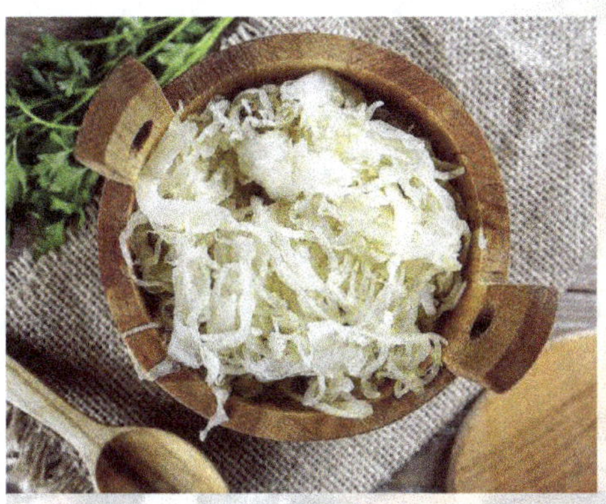

Ingredients:

- 1 medium-sized cabbage (green or red)

- 1 tablespoon of sea salt (non-iodized)

- Optional: Add juniper berries or caraway seeds for flavor

Procedures:

Prepare Cabbage:

- Remove outer leaves and set aside.

- Shred cabbage finely using a knife or a mandolin.

Massage Cabbage:

- In a large bowl, sprinkle salt over shredded cabbage.

- Massage and squeeze cabbage for about 10 minutes until it releases its juices.

Packaging in Jar:

- Pack the cabbage tightly into a clean, sterilized glass jar.

- Make sure the cabbage is completely immersed in its own juice.

Fermentation:

- Cover the jar with a cabbage leaf and a weight to keep the cabbage submerged.

- Seal the jar loosely to allow gas to escape.

- Place in a dark, room-temperature spot for 1-2 weeks.

Taste Test:

- After the fermentation period, taste the sauerkraut. If it's tangy enough for your liking, transfer to the fridge.

Time of Preparation:

- About 20 minutes for preparation.

- 1-2 weeks for fermentation.

Tips and Tricks:

- Use non-iodized salt to avoid hindering the fermentation process.

- Ensure all utensils and jars are thoroughly clean to prevent unwanted bacteria.

- Experiment with additional flavors like caraway seeds for a unique taste.

Nutritional Value per Serving (1 cup):

- Calories: 27

- Carbohydrates: 6g

- Fiber: 3g

- Vitamin C: 35% DV

- Probiotics: Lactic acid bacteria

Health Benefits:

- Rich in probiotics, promoting gut health.

- High in fiber, aiding digestion.

- Boosts immune system with vitamin C.

Packaging and Storing:

- Store in airtight jars in the refrigerator.

- Keeps well for several months.

Precautions:

- Ensure cleanliness during preparation to avoid contamination.

- Check for any signs of mold; discard if present.

- Introduce gradually if not accustomed to fermented foods.

Post-Caution:

- Enjoy sauerkraut in moderation to avoid excessive sodium intake.

- Consult a healthcare professional if you have concerns about probiotic consumption.

Homemade Yogurt for Gut Balance

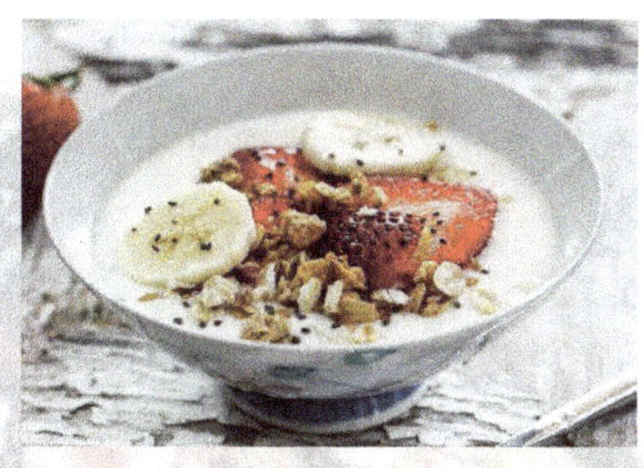

Ingredients:

- 1 quart (4 cups) of whole milk (organic, if possible)

- 2 tablespoons of plain yogurt with live active cultures (as a starter)

Procedures:

- Heat Milk: In a saucepan, heat the milk over medium heat until it reaches about 180°F (82°C). Stir occasionally to prevent scalding.

- Cool Milk: Let the milk cool to around 110°F (43°C). You can speed up the process by placing the saucepan in a cold-water bath.

- Inoculate with Starter: In a small bowl, mix the 2 tablespoons of plain yogurt with a small amount of the cooled milk.
- Add the yogurt mixture back into the saucepan and stir well.
- To incubate yogurt, transfer the milk mixture into jars or a sanitized container.
- Cover and keep the container in a warm place, maintaining a temperature of around 110°F (43°C), for 6-12 hours.
- Check Consistency: Once the yogurt has thickened, refrigerate for at least 2 hours to halt the fermentation process.
- Strain if a thicker Greek-style yogurt is desired.

Time of Preparation:

- Approximately 15 minutes for preparation.
- 6-12 hours for fermentation.

Tips and Tricks:

- Use a thermometer to monitor the temperature precisely.
- Keep the yogurt undisturbed during the incubation period.
- Use a clean container to avoid unwanted bacteria.

Nutritional Value per Serving (1 cup):

- Calories: 150
- Protein: 8g
- Fat: 8g
- Probiotics: Lactobacillus bulgaricus, Streptococcus thermophilus

Health Benefits:

- Supports gut health with probiotics.
- Rich in protein, calcium, and beneficial fats.
- May boost the immune system.

Packaging and Storing:

- Store yogurt in airtight containers in the refrigerator.
- Consume within 1-2 weeks for optimal freshness.

Precautions:

- Ensure utensils and containers are clean to prevent contamination.
- Avoid using ultra-pasteurized milk, as it may affect the fermentation process.

Post-Caution:

- If experiencing digestive discomfort, start with small amounts of yogurt.
- Consult a healthcare professional if you have lactose intolerance or dairy allergies.

Fermented Pickles to Boost Digestion

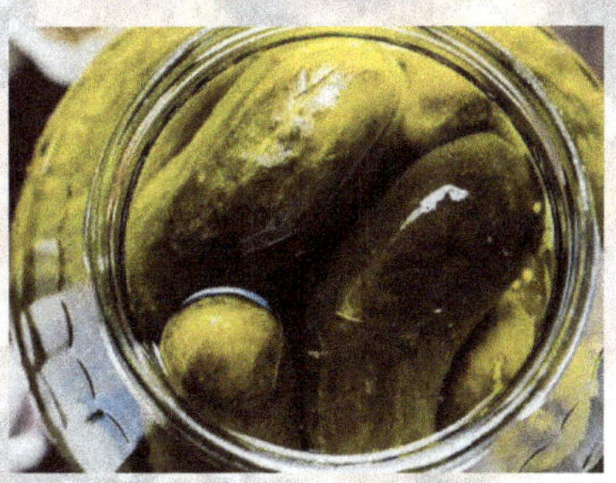

Ingredients:

- 2 pounds of pickling cucumbers
- 1-2 heads of fresh dill
- 4 cloves of garlic, peeled

- 1 tablespoon of whole black peppercorns
- 1 tablespoon of coriander seeds
- 2 tablespoons of sea salt
- 4 cups of water (non-chlorinated)

Procedures:

- Prepare Cucumbers: Wash and trim the ends of the cucumbers. Cut into desired shapes.
- Create Brine: In a saucepan, dissolve sea salt in water, creating the brine solution. Let it cool.
- Pack Jars: In clean, sterilized jars, layer cucumbers, fresh dill, garlic, peppercorns, and coriander seeds.
- Pour Brine: Pour the cooled brine over the cucumber mixture, ensuring all ingredients are submerged.
- Fermentation: Seal jars loosely to allow gases to escape. Place in a dark, room-temperature spot for 3-5 days.
- Check Pickles: Taste the pickles; once they reach the desired level of fermentation, move jars to the refrigerator to slow down the process.

Time of Preparation:

- Approximately 20 minutes for preparation.
- 3-5 days for fermentation.

Tips and Tricks:

- Use pickling cucumbers for crispiness.
- Ensure the cucumbers stay submerged in the brine to avoid spoilage.
- Adjust flavorings to personal preference.

Nutritional Value per Serving (1 pickle):

- Calories: 5

- Sodium: 300mg

- Probiotics: Lactic acid bacteria

Health Benefits:

- Enhances digestion with probiotics.

- Low-calorie snack.

- Provides a source of electrolytes.

Packaging and Storing:

- Store in airtight jars in the refrigerator.

- Pickles can be enjoyed for several weeks.

Precautions:

- Use non-chlorinated water to avoid inhibiting fermentation.

- Ensure jars and utensils are thoroughly clean.

Post-Caution:

- Try tinier doses at first to prevent upset stomach.

- Monitor for any signs of spoilage; discard if mold or off-putting odor is detected.

Gut Healing Chicken Soup

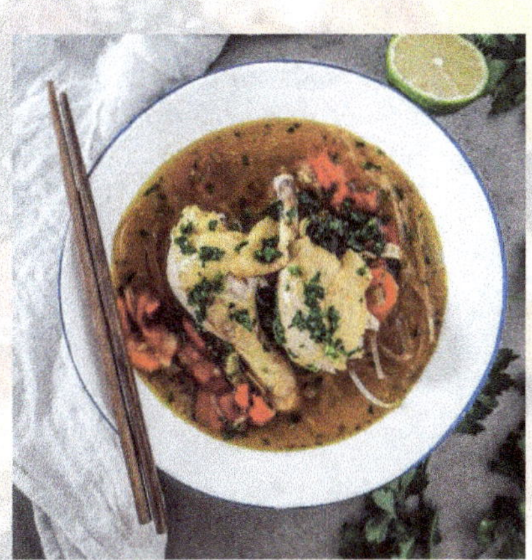

Ingredients:

- 1 whole organic chicken, preferably free-range

- 8 cups bone broth

- 2 carrots, peeled and sliced

- 2 celery stalks, chopped
- 1 onion, diced
- 3 cloves garlic, minced
- 1-inch ginger, grated
- 1 cup kale, chopped
- 1 tablespoon turmeric powder
- 1 teaspoon sea salt
- 1/2 teaspoon black pepper
- Fresh parsley for garnish

Procedure:

- Transfer the entire chicken into a big pot, pour in the bone broth, and heat it until it boils. After lowering the heat, simmer it for thirty minutes.

After eliminating any froth that floats to the top, include the carrots, celery, onion, ginger, and garlic. Simmer for another half hour more.

- Remove any foam that rises to the surface and add carrots, celery, onion, garlic, and ginger. Simmer for another half hour more.
- Add turmeric, sea salt, and black pepper. Stir well and simmer for another 15-20 minutes until the chicken is fully cooked.
- Remove the chicken from the pot, shred the meat, and return it to the soup. Add chopped kale and simmer for an extra 5-10 minutes until the kale is tender.
- Adjust seasoning if necessary. Serve hot, garnished with fresh parsley.

Time of Preparation:

- Approximately 1 hour and 30 minutes.

Tips and Tricks:

- Use organic and free-range chicken for enhanced flavor and nutritional value.

- Add a splash of apple cider vinegar while simmering the chicken to extract more nutrients from the bones.

- Customize the vegetables based on personal preferences for added variety.

Nutritional Value (per serving):

- Calories: 200

- Protein: 25g

- Carbohydrates: 10g

- Fat: 8g

- Fiber: 3g

Health Benefits:

- Rich in collagen and gelatin, promoting gut health.

- Turmeric and ginger provide anti-inflammatory properties.

- Nutrient-dense vegetables contribute to overall well-being.

Packaging and Storing:

- Let the soup cool fully before putting it in sealed jars. For extended storage, freeze or refrigerate for up to four days. Reheat on the burner, but gently.

Precautions:

- Ensure chicken is fully cooked to avoid foodborne illnesses. Consult a healthcare professional if you have allergies or specific dietary concerns.

Post-Caution:

- Listen to your body's response to the soup. If any adverse reactions occur, discontinue consumption and seek medical advice. Always get the advice of a medical expert before making any dietary changes.

Butternut Squash & Carrot Immunity Soup

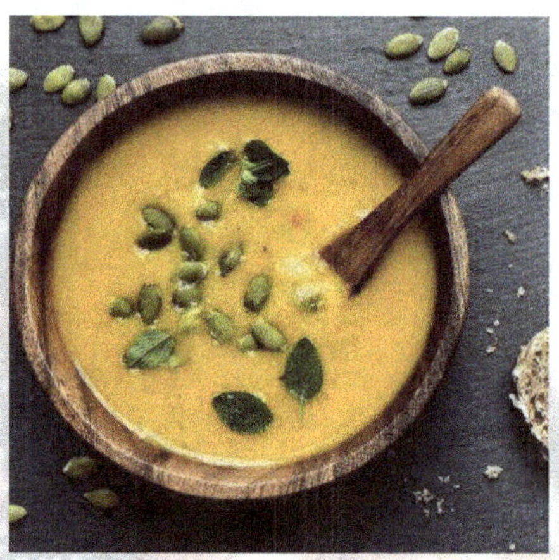

Ingredients:

- One medium butternut squash that has been diced, skinned, and seeded 3 large carrots, peeled and sliced

- 1 onion, diced

- 3 cloves garlic, minced

- 1 tablespoon olive oil

- 6 cups vegetable broth

- 1 teaspoon ground turmeric

- 1 teaspoon ground cumin

- 1/2 teaspoon cinnamon

- Salt and pepper to taste

- Fresh cilantro for garnish

Procedure:

- Add the onion and garlic to a large pot and sauté in olive oil until they soften.

- Add butternut squash and carrots, stirring for 5 minutes.

- Pour in vegetable broth, turmeric, cumin, cinnamon, salt, and pepper. Bring to a boil, then reduce heat and simmer for 20-25 minutes until vegetables are tender.

- Puree the soup with an immersion blender until it's smooth. As an alternative, move batches to a blender, purée them, and then put them back in the pot.

- Adjust seasoning if needed. Serve hot, garnished with fresh cilantro.

Time of Preparation:

- Approximately 40 minutes.

Tips and Tricks:

- Roast the butternut squash for added depth of flavor.

- Add a small amount of cream or coconut milk for a creamier texture.

- For a creamier texture, add a splash of coconut milk or cream.

Nutritional Value (per serving):

- Calories: 150

- Protein: 2g

- Carbohydrates: 35g

- Fat: 1g

- Fiber: 6g

Health Benefits:

- Butternut squash and carrots provide beta-carotene, supporting immune function.
- Turmeric and cumin have anti-inflammatory properties.
- Rich in vitamins A and C for overall immune system support.

Packaging and Storing:

- Allow the soup to cool before transferring it to airtight containers. Refrigerate for up to 3-4 days or freeze for longer storage. Reheat on the stove or in the microwave.

Precautions:

- Ensure vegetables are thoroughly cooked to avoid digestive discomfort. Adjust spice levels according to personal tolerance. If allergies are a concern, consult with a healthcare professional.

Post-Caution:

- Monitor your body's response to the soup. If any adverse reactions occur, discontinue consumption and seek medical advice. Always consult with a healthcare professional for personalized dietary recommendations.

Creamy Zucchini Soup for Gut Nourishment

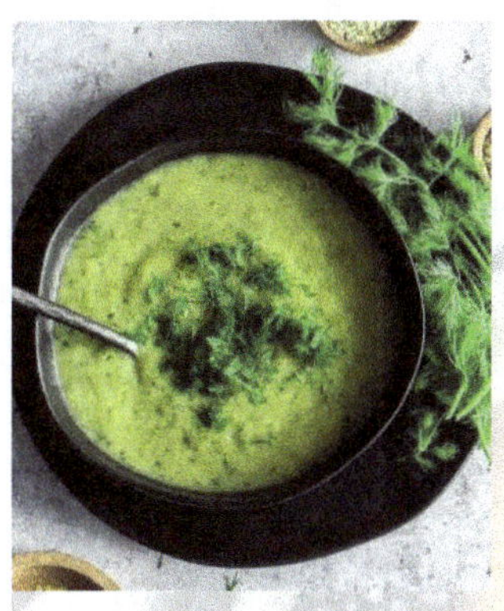

Ingredients:

- 4 medium-sized zucchinis, sliced
- 1 onion, chopped
- 2 cloves garlic, minced
- 2 tablespoons olive oil
- 4 cups vegetable broth
- 1 potato, peeled and diced
- 1 teaspoon dried thyme
- Salt and pepper to taste
- 1/2 cup Greek yogurt or coconut milk (for creaminess)
- Fresh chives for garnish

Procedure:

- In a large pot, sauté onion and garlic in olive oil until translucent.
- Add zucchinis, potato, thyme, salt, and pepper. Stir for 5 minutes.
- Pour in vegetable broth, bring to a boil, then reduce heat and simmer for 20-25 minutes until vegetables are tender.
- Use an immersion blender to puree the soup until smooth. Add Greek yogurt or coconut milk, blend until creamy.
- Adjust seasoning if necessary. Serve hot, garnished with fresh chives.

Time of Preparation:

- Approximately 40 minutes.

Tips and Tricks:

- Use young zucchinis for a smoother texture.
- Add a pinch of nutmeg for an extra layer of flavor.
- Experiment with different herbs to customize the taste.

Nutritional Value (per serving):

- Calories: 120
- Protein: 3g
- Carbohydrates: 18g
- Fat: 5g
- Fiber: 4g

Health Benefits:

- Zucchinis are rich in fiber, promoting gut health.
- Greek yogurt provides probiotics for digestive support.
- Olive oil contributes healthy fats.

Packaging and Storing:

- Allow the soup to cool before transferring it to airtight containers. Refrigerate for up to 3-4 days or freeze for longer storage. Reheat on the stove or in the microwave.

Precautions:

- Be cautious with the addition of salt; it's easier to add more later. If lactose intolerant, consider dairy-free alternatives.

Post-Caution:

- Monitor your body's response to the soup. If any adverse reactions occur, discontinue consumption and seek medical advice. Always consult with a healthcare professional for personalized dietary recommendations.

3

Protein-Rich Main Dishes

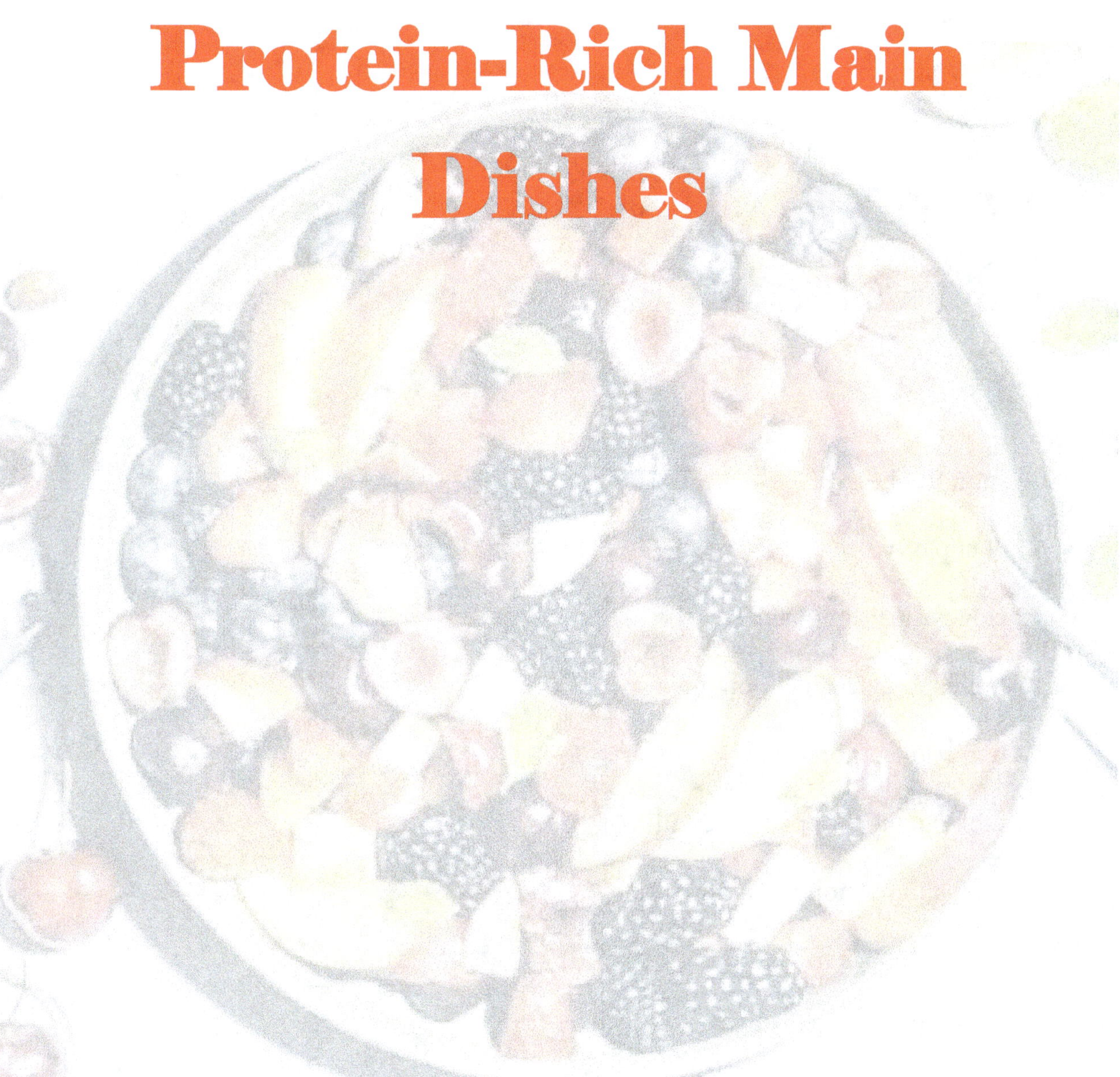

35 | GAPS COOKBOOK FOR GUT HEALTH

Baked Salmon with Lemon and Herbs

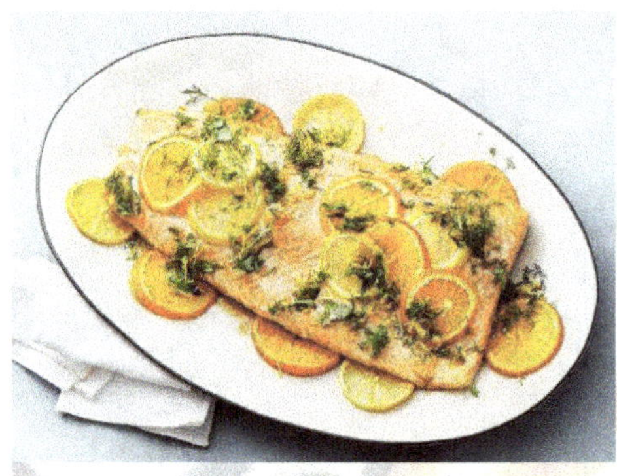

Ingredients:

- 4 salmon fillets

- 1/4 cup olive oil

- 2 cloves garlic, minced

- 1 tablespoon fresh lemon juice

- 1 teaspoon lemon zest

- 1 tablespoon chopped fresh dill

- 1 tablespoon chopped fresh parsley

- Salt and pepper to taste

- Lemon slices for garnish

Procedure:

- Turn the oven on to 375° F, or 190° C.

  Arrange the salmon fillets onto a parchment paper-lined baking sheet.

  Combine the olive oil, minced garlic, lemon zest, juice, parsley, dill, and salt & pepper in a small bowl.

  Make sure the salmon fillets are evenly coated by gently brushing them with the herb mixture.

  Top each fillet with a slice of lemon for extra taste.

  Bake the salmon for 15 to 20 minutes, or until it is cooked through and flake readily when tested with a fork.

- Garnish with additional fresh herbs and lemon slices before serving.

Time of Preparation:

- Approximately 25 minutes (including prep and baking time).

Tips and Tricks:

- Pat the salmon dry before applying the herb mixture for better adherence.

- Take into account the thickness of your salmon fillets when adjusting the cooking time.

- For added flavor, marinate the salmon in the herb mixture for 30 minutes before baking.

Nutritional Value per Serving:

- Calories: 300

- Protein: 25g

- Fat: 20g

- Carbohydrates: 2g

- Fiber: 1g

Health Benefits:

- Packed with omega-3 fatty acids, which support heart health.

- High protein content supports muscle development.

- Lemon and herbs provide antioxidants and boost immune function.

Packaging and Storing:

- Keep leftovers refrigerated for up to two days in an airtight container.

- For longer storage, freeze the baked salmon, ensuring it's well-wrapped to prevent freezer burn.

Precautions:

- Ensure the salmon reaches an internal temperature of 145°F (63°C) to guarantee it's fully cooked.

- If allergic to any ingredients, substitute accordingly.

- Use caution when handling hot baking sheets and pans.

Post-Caution:

- Any leftovers left out for longer than two hours should be thrown out.

- Reheat leftovers thoroughly before consumption to prevent foodborne illnesses.

Grass-Fed Beef Stir-Fry with Vegetables

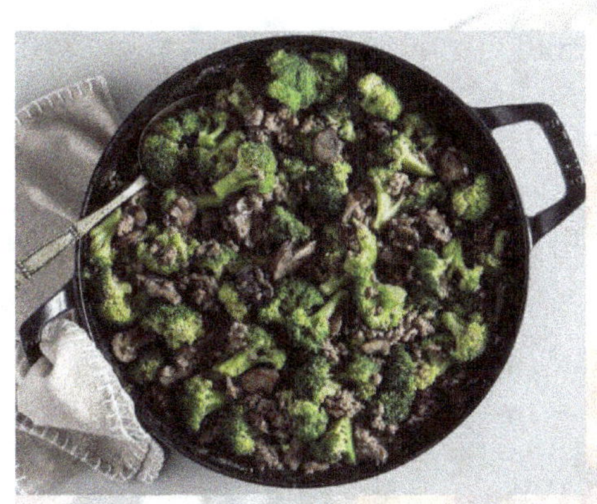

Ingredients:

- 1pound grass-fed beef sirloin, thinly sliced

- A couple of teaspoons of soy sauce (or, for a gluten-free option, tamari)

- 1 tablespoon oyster sauce

- 1 tablespoon sesame oil

- 2 cloves garlic, minced

- 1 tablespoon fresh ginger, grated

- 2 tablespoons vegetable oil

- 1 broccoli crown, cut into florets

- 1 bell pepper, thinly sliced

- 1 carrot, julienned

- 1 cup snap peas, ends trimmed

- 2 green onions, sliced

- Sesame seeds for garnish

Procedure:

- Combine oyster sauce, sesame oil, and soy sauce in a bowl. Let the beef slices marinate in this marinade for a minimum of fifteen minutes. In a wok or big skillet, heat the vegetable oil over medium-high heat. Add the grated ginger and minced garlic, and sauté for 30 seconds, or until fragrant. Stir-fry the marinated beef pieces until they are cooked through and browned. Take the steak out of the wok and place it aside.

- In the same wok, add more oil if needed and stir-fry broccoli, bell pepper, carrot, and snap peas until vegetables are crisp-tender.

- Return the cooked beef to the wok, add sliced green onions, and toss to combine.

- Garnish with sesame seeds before serving.

Time of Preparation:

- About half an hour (including time for marinating and frying).

Tips and Tricks:

- Partially freeze the beef for easier slicing.

- Use a high smoke point oil like peanut or grapeseed oil for stir-frying.

- Cut vegetables uniformly for even cooking.

Nutritional Value per Serving:

- Calories: 350

- Protein: 25g

- Fat: 20g

- Carbohydrates: 15g

- Fiber: 5g

Health Benefits:

- Grass-fed beef is rich in omega-3 fatty acids and has higher levels of antioxidants.

- Vegetables are a great source of vitamins and minerals.

- Ginger and garlic may have anti-inflammatory and immune-boosting properties.

Packaging and Storing:

- Keep leftovers refrigerated for up to three days in an airtight container. Reheat in a skillet or microwave until thoroughly heated.

Precautions:

- Ensure beef reaches a safe internal temperature of 145°F (63°C).

- Be cautious when working with a hot wok or skillet.

- Check for any food allergies before using soy or oyster sauce.

Post-Caution:

- Discard any perishable leftovers that have been left at room temperature for more than 2 hours.

- To avoid contamination, handle and store food safely.

Turkey and Sweet Potato Casserole

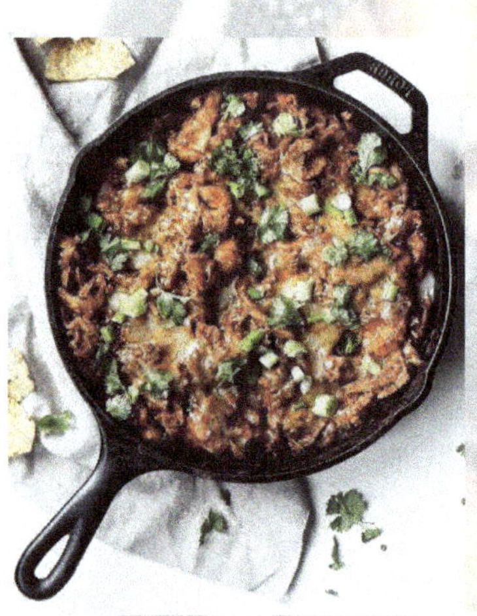

Ingredients:

- 1 pound ground turkey

- 2 medium sweet potatoes, peeled and thinly sliced

- 1 onion, finely chopped

- 2 cloves garlic, minced

- 1 cup frozen peas

- 1 cup turkey or chicken broth

- 1/2 cup milk (or dairy-free alternative)

- 2 tablespoons flour (or gluten-free flour)

- 2 tablespoons olive oil

- 1 teaspoon dried thyme

- Salt and pepper to taste

- 1 cup shredded cheddar cheese (optional)

- Fresh parsley for garnish

Procedure:

- Preheat the oven to 375°F (190°C).

- Heat olive oil in a big skillet over medium heat. Add the minced garlic and onions, and cook until they soften.

- Add ground turkey and cook until browned. Drain excess fat if needed.

- Sprinkle flour over the turkey mixture, stir to combine.

- Gradually add broth, stirring continuously to avoid lumps. Add milk, thyme, salt, and pepper. Simmer until the mixture thickens.

- Layer half of the sweet potato slices in a greased casserole dish, followed by the turkey mixture, frozen peas, and the remaining sweet potato slices.

- Cover the dish with foil and bake for 40-45 minutes, or until sweet potatoes are tender.

- Optionally, sprinkle shredded cheddar cheese on top during the last 10 minutes of baking.

- Garnish with fresh parsley before serving.

Time of Preparation:

- Approximately 1 hour (including prep and baking time).

Tips and Tricks:

- Use a mandoline slicer for uniform sweet potato slices.

- Adjust seasoning to taste preferences.

- Personalize by including your preferred herbs or spices.

Nutritional Value per Serving:

- Calories: 350

- Protein: 20g

- Fat: 15g

- Carbohydrates: 30g

- Fiber: 5g

Health Benefits:

- Sweet potatoes are abundant in antioxidants, fiber, and vitamins.

- Turkey provides lean protein essential for muscle health.

- Peas add fiber and essential nutrients.

Packaging and Storing:

- Allow the casserole to cool before storing in an airtight container in the refrigerator for up to 3 days.

- Reheat in the microwave or oven until thoroughly warmed.

Precautions:

- Ensure ground turkey is cooked to an internal temperature of 165°F (74°C).

- Check for food allergies before using flour or cheese.

Post-Caution:

- Any leftovers left out for longer than two hours should be thrown out.

- Use safe food handling practices to avoid contamination.

4
Vegetarian Delights

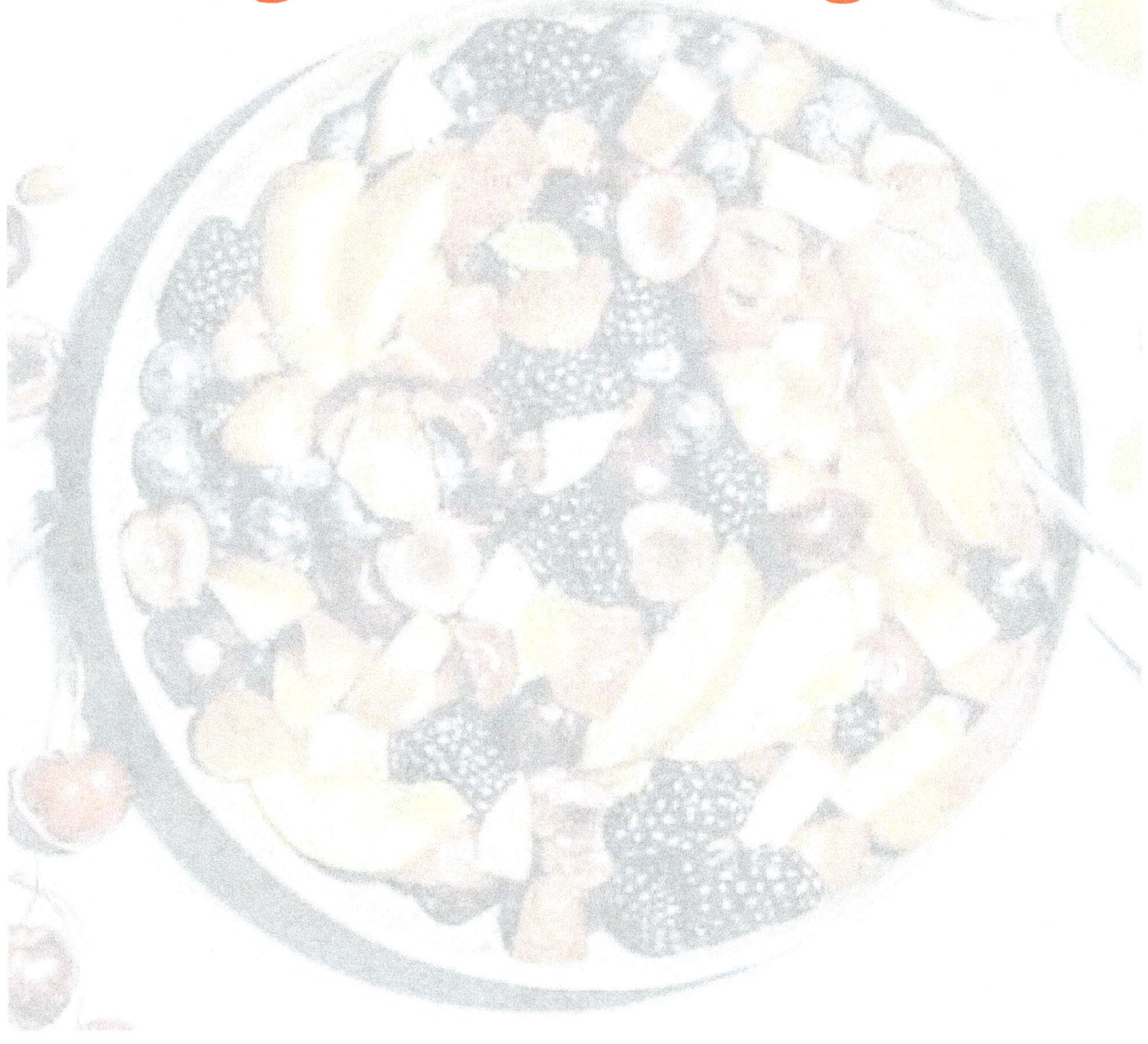

Quinoa and Roasted Veggie Bowl

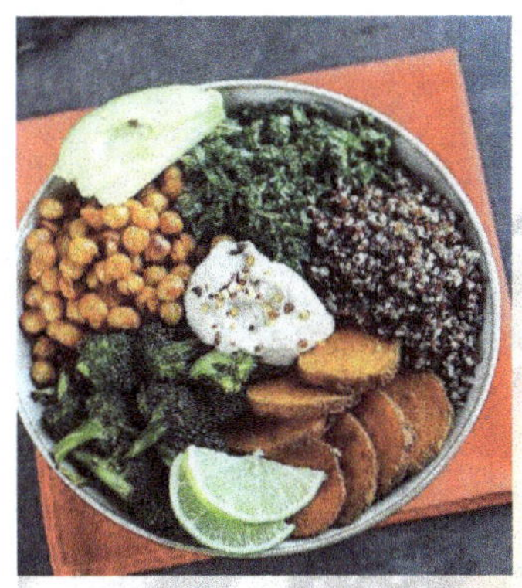

Procedures:

Procedures:

- Rinse quinoa thoroughly under cold water.

- Place the quinoa and two cups of water in a saucepan. After bringing to a boil, lower the heat, cover, and simmer until the water is absorbed, around 15 to 20 minutes.

- Preheat the oven to 400°F (200°C).

- In a bowl, toss mixed vegetables with olive oil, garlic powder, onion powder, dried oregano, salt, and pepper.

- Spread seasoned veggies on a baking sheet and roast for 20-25 minutes, or until they are tender and slightly browned.

Ingredients:

- 1 cup quinoa

- 2 cups of mixed veggies, such as cherry tomatoes, bell peppers, and zucchini

- 1 tablespoon olive oil

- 1 teaspoon garlic powder

- 1 teaspoon onion powder

- 1 teaspoon dried oregano

- Salt and pepper to taste

- 1/4 cup feta cheese (optional)

- Fresh parsley for garnish

- Fluff cooked quinoa with a fork and distribute it among serving bowls.
- Top quinoa with the roasted veggies, sprinkle with feta cheese (if using), and garnish with fresh parsley.

Time of Preparation:

- Approximately 40-45 minutes.

Tips and Tricks:

- Customize veggies based on preference.
- Drizzle balsamic glaze or tahini for extra flavor.
- Add grilled chicken or chickpeas for added protein.

Nutritional Value per Serving:

- Quinoa provides essential amino acids, fiber, and minerals.
- Vegetables offer vitamins and antioxidants.
- Feta contributes calcium and protein.

Health Benefits:

- High in protein, promoting muscle health.
- Rich in fiber, aiding digestion and weight management.
- Packed with vitamins for overall well-being.

Packaging and Storing:

- Keep refrigerated in sealed containers for a maximum of three days.

Reheat on the stove or in the microwave.

Precautions:

- Check for allergies to quinoa or specific vegetables.
- Adjust salt and seasoning based on dietary restrictions.

Post-Caution:

- Ensure proper storage to prevent spoilage.
- Monitor portion sizes for dietary balance.

Lentil and Spinach Stew

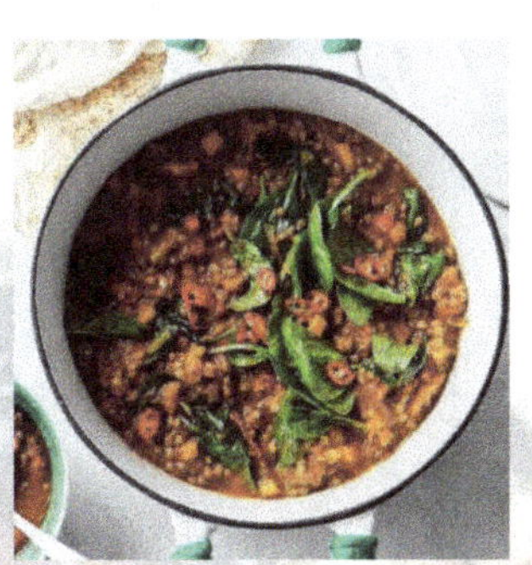

Ingredients:

- 1 cup dry green or brown lentils
- 1 onion, diced
- 3 cloves garlic, minced
- 2 carrots, sliced
- 2 celery stalks, chopped
- 1 can (14 oz) diced tomatoes
- 4 cups vegetable broth
- 1 teaspoon ground cumin
- 1 teaspoon smoked paprika
- 1/2 teaspoon ground coriander
- Salt and pepper to taste
- 4 cups fresh spinach
- 1 tablespoon olive oil

- Lemon wedges for serving (optional)

Procedures:

- Lentils should be rinsed with cold water and left aside.

Add the onion and garlic to a large pot and sauté in olive oil until they soften.

Include the lentils, celery, and carrots in the pot. Mix everything together.

Add the chopped tomatoes, vegetable broth, coriander, cumin, smoked paprika, salt, and pepper.

After bringing the mixture to a boil, lower the heat, and simmer the lentils for 25 to 30 minutes, or until they become soft.

Add the fresh spinach and stir until it wilts.

Serve hot with lemon wedges and adjust spice as needed.

Time of Preparation:

- Approximately 40-45 minutes.

Tips and Tricks:

- Use red lentils for a quicker cooking time.
- Enhance flavor with a splash of balsamic vinegar.
- Add some fresh herbs, like parsley or cilantro, as a garnish.

Nutritional Value per Serving:

- Lentils provide protein, fiber, and essential minerals.
- Spinach offers vitamins A, C, and K.
- Low in fat and high in nutrients.

Health Benefits:

- Supports heart health with fiber and low-fat content.

- Rich in iron and folate, benefiting blood health.

- Aids digestion and promotes weight management.

Packaging and Storing:

- For up to three days, store in the refrigerator in sealed containers.

  Reheat using a stovetop or microwave.

Precautions:

- Be cautious with sodium levels in vegetable broth.

- Check for allergies to lentils or specific vegetables.

Post-Caution:

- Ensure proper storage to maintain freshness.

- Monitor portion sizes for dietary balance.

Cauliflower Rice Pilaf for Gut Health

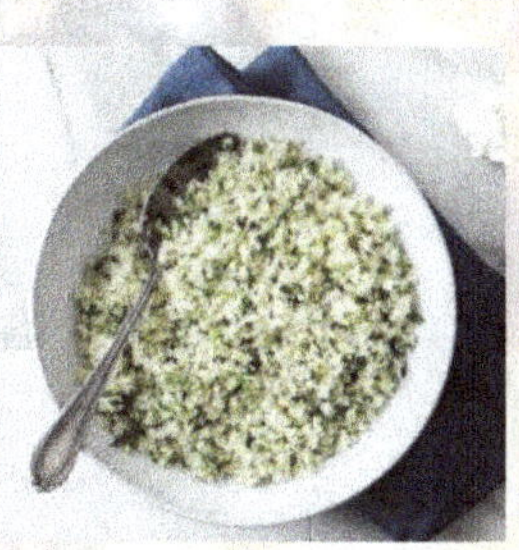

Ingredients:

- 1 medium cauliflower head, grated into "rice"

- 2 tablespoons olive oil

- 1 onion, finely chopped

- 2 cloves garlic, minced

- 1 carrot, grated

- 1 cup frozen peas

- 1/4 cup chopped fresh parsley

- 1 teaspoon ground cumin

- 1/2 teaspoon turmeric powder

- Salt and pepper to taste

- 1/4 cup toasted almonds, chopped (optional)

Procedures:

- Grate the cauliflower into small rice-sized pieces using a food processor or box grater.

- In a large pan, heat olive oil over medium heat and sauté onions until translucent.

- Add minced garlic and cook for another minute.

- Stir in cauliflower rice, grated carrot, frozen peas, ground cumin, turmeric, salt, and pepper.

- Cook for 5-7 minutes, stirring occasionally, until cauliflower rice is tender but not mushy.

- Mix in chopped parsley and toasted almonds if using.

- Adjust seasoning if necessary and serve warm.

Time of Preparation:

- Approximately 20-25 minutes.

Tips and Tricks

- Ensure cauliflower is dry before grating to avoid excess moisture.

- Experiment with additional herbs and spices for flavor variation.

- Add a squeeze of lemon juice for a citrusy twist.

Nutritional Value per Serving:

- Low in calories, suitable for weight management.

- Cauliflower provides fiber, aiding digestion.
- Turmeric and cumin have anti-inflammatory properties.

Health Benefits:

- Promotes gut health with fiber and beneficial nutrients.
- Supports weight loss with low-calorie content.
- Anti-inflammatory effects from turmeric.

Packaging and Storing:

- For up to three days, store in the refrigerator in sealed containers.

  Reheat using a stovetop or microwave.

Precautions:

- Check for allergies to cauliflower or specific spices.
- Monitor portion sizes for those with digestive sensitivities.

Post-Caution:

- Ensure proper storage to prevent spoilage.
- Incorporate into a balanced diet for optimal gut health.

5

GAPS-Friendly Snacks

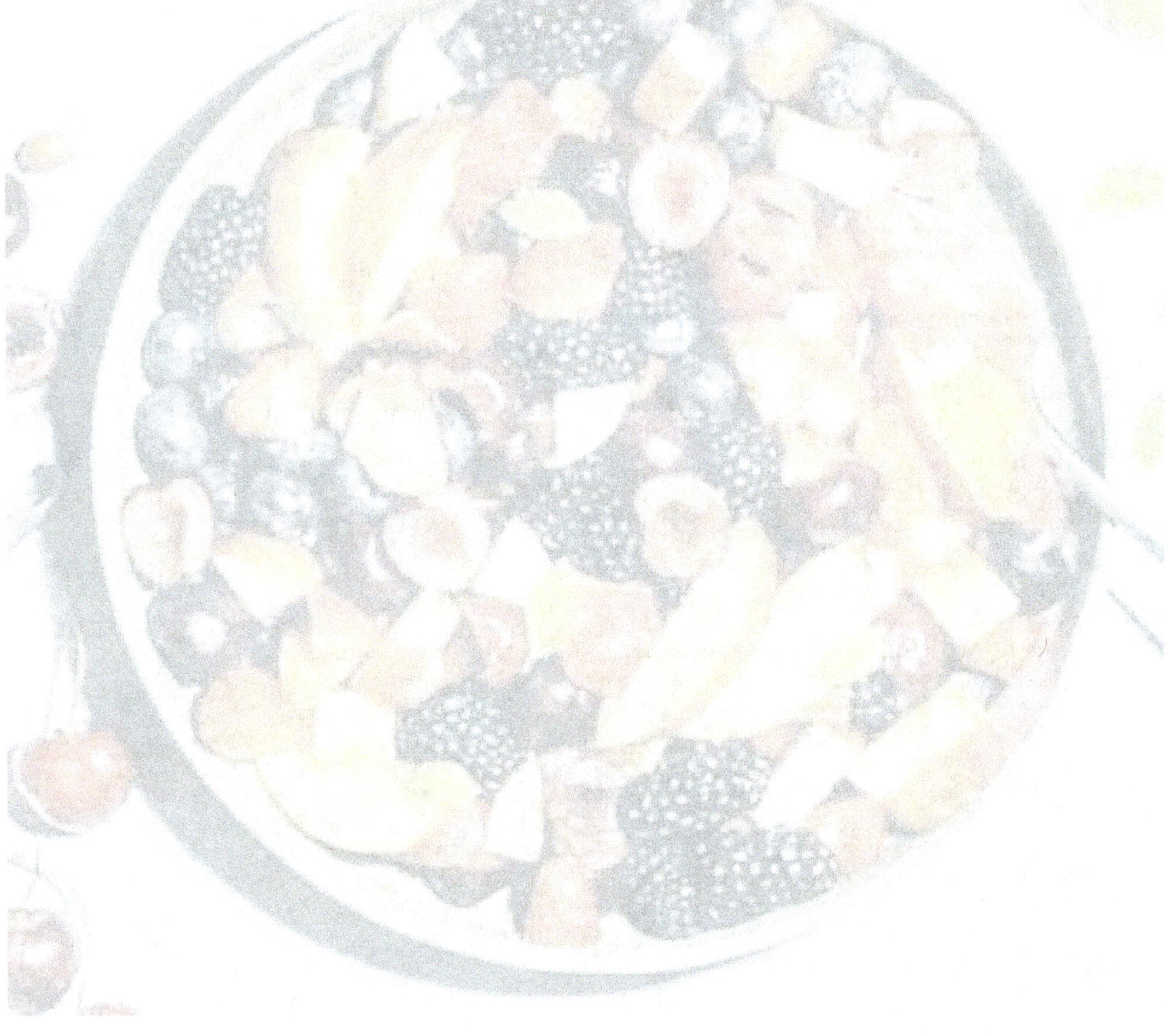

Avocado and Salsa Dip

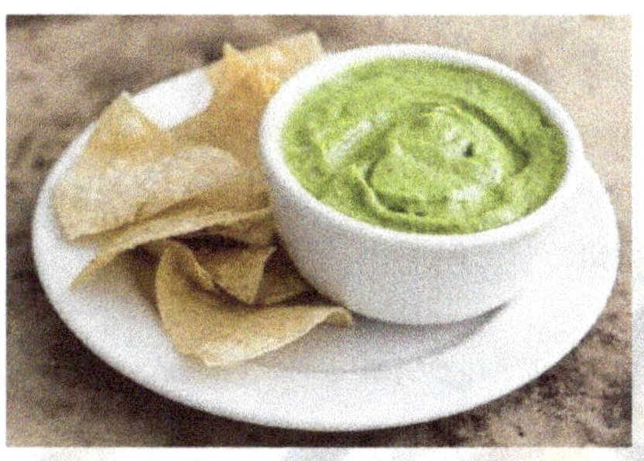

Ingredients:

- 2 ripe avocados
- 1 cup diced tomatoes
- 1/2 cup finely chopped red onion
- 1/4 cup chopped cilantro
- 1 jalapeño, seeded and minced
- 2 cloves garlic, minced
- Juice of 1 lime
- Salt and pepper to taste

Procedure:

- Prepare Avocados: Cut avocados in half, remove the pit, and scoop the flesh into a bowl.
- Mash Avocados: Mash avocados using a fork or potato masher until smooth or leave it chunky for texture.
- Combine Ingredients: Add diced tomatoes, red onion, cilantro, jalapeño, and minced garlic to the mashed avocados.
- Season: Squeeze lime juice over the mixture and add salt and pepper to taste. Mix well.
- Chill: Refrigerate the dip for at least 30 minutes to allow flavors to meld.

Time of Preparation:

- Approximately 15-20 minutes

Tips and Tricks:

- Choose ripe avocados for a creamier texture.

- Adjust spice level by adding or omitting jalapeño seeds.
- For extra freshness, add chopped mango or pineapple.
- Cover the dip with plastic wrap, pressing it directly onto the surface to prevent browning.

Nutritional Value (per serving, based on a typical 1/4 cup serving):

- Calories: 100
- Fat: 8g
- Saturated Fat: 1g
- Cholesterol: 0mg
- Sodium: 50mg
- Carbohydrates: 7g
- Fiber: 4g
- Sugars: 1g
- Protein: 1g

Health Benefits:

- Rich in heart-healthy monounsaturated fats from avocados.
- Provides a good dose of fiber, promoting digestive health.
- Loaded with vitamins and antioxidants from tomatoes, onions, and cilantro.

Packaging and Storing:

- Keep refrigerated in an airtight container.
- To prevent browning, press plastic wrap directly onto the dip's surface.
- Consume within 2 days for optimal freshness.

Precautions:

- Be cautious while handling jalapeños; consider wearing gloves and avoid touching your face.

- Check the avocado's ripeness to ensure the dip's creamy consistency.

Post-Caution:

- If the dip turns slightly brown due to avocado oxidation, it's still safe to eat; just stir before serving.

- Adjust salt and lime if needed before serving leftovers.

Almond Flour Crackers

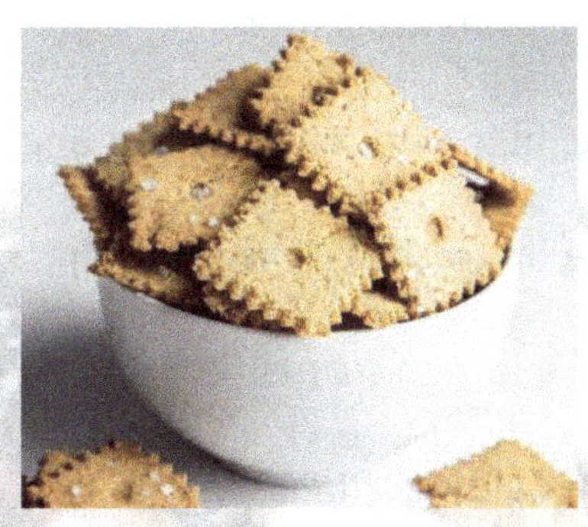

Ingredients:

- 2 cups almond flour

- 1 egg

- 1 tablespoon olive oil

- 1/2 teaspoon salt

- 1/2 teaspoon garlic powder

- 1/2 teaspoon dried rosemary (optional)

- 1/4 teaspoon baking soda

- Sesame seeds for topping (optional)

Procedure:

- Preheat Oven: Preheat your oven to 350°F (175°C).

- Mix Dry Ingredients: In a bowl, combine almond flour, salt, garlic powder, and baking soda.

- Add Wet Ingredients: Add the egg and olive oil to the dry ingredients. Mix until a dough forms.

- Roll Out Dough: Place the dough between two sheets of parchment paper and roll it out thinly.

- Cut into Shapes: Use a knife or cookie cutter to cut the rolled-out dough into desired cracker shapes.

- Transfer to Baking Sheet: Carefully transfer the cut crackers to a parchment-lined baking sheet.

- Optional Toppings: Sprinkle sesame seeds or dried rosemary on top for added flavor.

- Bake: Bake for 10 to 12 minutes, or until the edges are golden brown, in an oven that has been warmed.

- Cool and Break Apart: Allow the crackers to cool on the baking sheet, then break them apart along the cut lines.

Time of Preparation:

- Approximately 25 minutes

Tips and Tricks:

- Ensure the almond flour is finely ground for a smoother texture.

- Experiment with different spices like onion powder or paprika for varied flavors.

- To achieve a more crunchy texture, roll the dough thinner.

Nutritional Value (per serving, based on a typical 1-ounce serving):

- Calories: 140

- Fat: 12g

- Saturated Fat: 1g

- Cholesterol: 16mg

- Sodium: 130mg

- Carbohydrates: 4g

- Fiber: 2g

- Sugars: 0g

- Protein: 5g

Health Benefits:

- High in healthy fats from almond flour, promoting heart health.

- Gluten-free alternative suitable for those with gluten sensitivity.

- Rich in vitamin E and antioxidants from almonds.

Packaging and Storing:

- Retain at room temperature in a sealed container.

- To maintain crispiness, include a small piece of bread or a silica gel packet in the container.

Precautions:

- Monitor baking closely to prevent over-browning.

- Adjust salt and spices according to personal preferences.

Post-Caution:

- If crackers lose crispiness, reheat in the oven for a few minutes.

- Consider adding fresh herbs or cheese when serving for extra flavor.

Gut-Supporting Energy Bites

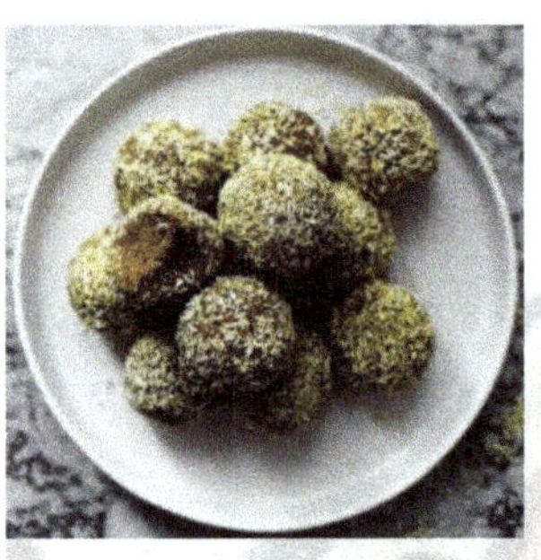

Ingredients:

- 1 cup rolled oats
- 1/2 cup almond butter
- 1/3 cup honey or maple syrup
- 1/4 cup ground flaxseed
- 1/4 cup chia seeds
- 1 teaspoon vanilla extract
- 1/2 teaspoon ground cinnamon
- 1/2 cup shredded coconut (optional, for coating)
- 1/4 cup chopped nuts (e.g., almonds, walnuts)

Procedure:

- Combine Ingredients: In a bowl, mix rolled oats, almond butter, honey, ground flaxseed, chia seeds, vanilla extract, and ground cinnamon.

- Add Nuts: Fold in the chopped nuts for added crunch and nutritional value.

- Chill Mixture: Place the mixture in the refrigerator for about 30 minutes to make it easier to handle.

- Shape into Bites: Take small portions and roll the mixture into bite-sized balls using your hands.

- Optional Coating: If desired, roll the energy bites in shredded coconut for an extra layer of flavor and texture.

- Refrigerate: Store the energy bites in the refrigerator for at least one hour to set.

Time of Preparation:

- Approximately 15-20 minutes

Tips and Tricks:

- Customize with your favorite nuts, seeds, or dried fruits for variety.
- Adjust sweetness by modifying the amount of honey or using alternatives like maple syrup.
- For a more intense flavor, toast the rolled oats before mixing.

Nutritional Value (per serving, based on a typical 2-bite serving):

- Calories: 180
- Fat: 10g
- Saturated Fat: 1g
- Cholesterol: 0mg
- Sodium: 10mg
- Carbohydrates: 20g
- Fiber: 4g
- Sugars: 9g
- Protein: 5g

Health Benefits:

- Rich in fiber from oats, flaxseed, and chia seeds, supporting gut health.
- Almond butter has magnesium, vitamin E, and good lipids.
- Chia seeds offer omega-3 fatty acids, promoting heart health.

Packaging and Storing:

- Store in the refrigerator in an airtight container, making sure to separate the layers with parchment paper to avoid adhering.
- Can be frozen for longer storage; thaw before consuming.

Precautions:

- Individuals with nut allergies should choose nut-free alternatives.
- Watch the sweetness level to align with personal preferences and dietary needs.

Post-Caution:

- Energy bites can soften at room temperature, so store and serve chilled.
- Experiment with different coatings or drizzles for added variety.

6

Probiotic Beverages

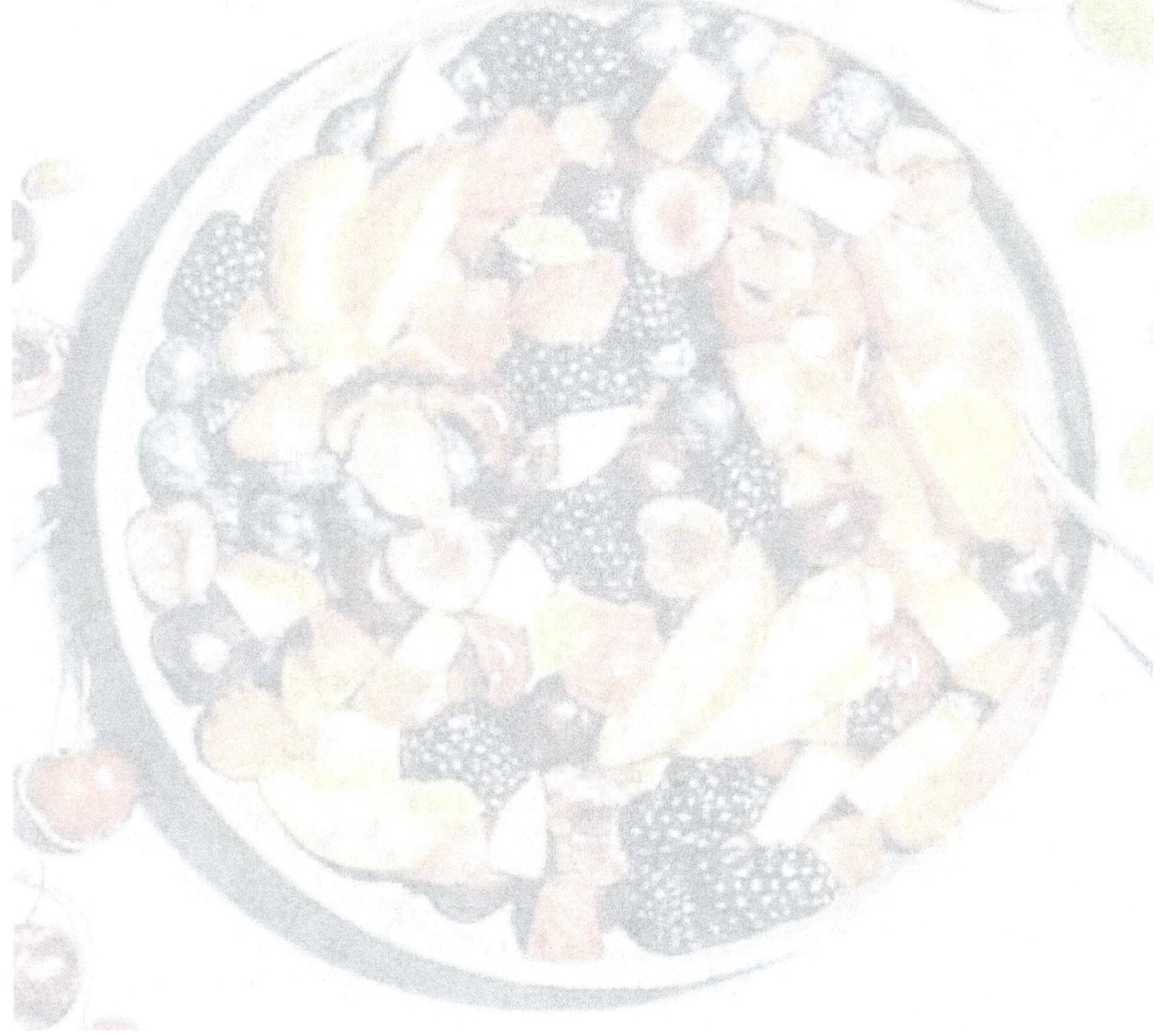

Ginger Kombucha Elixir

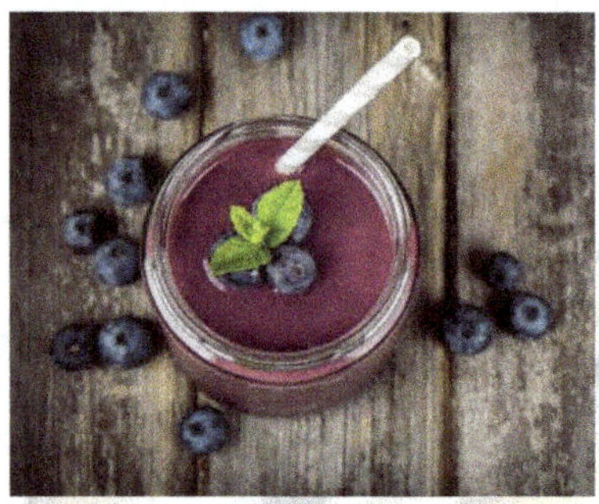

Ingredients:

- 1 SCOBY (Symbiotic Culture Of Bacteria and Yeast)
- 1 cup of sugar (for fermentation)
- 4-6 black or green tea bags
- 1 gallon of filtered water
- One cup of starting tea (either store-bought kombucha or from a prior batch)
- 1 cup of fresh ginger, sliced or grated
- Glass jars for brewing and storing
- Cloth or paper towel for covering the jars
- Rubber bands or string to secure the covering

Procedure:

- The sweet tea can be made by boiling four cups of water and steeping the tea bags for ten to fifteen minutes. Stir in the sugar and mix until it dissolves. When the tea cools to room temperature, let it.
- Ingredients should be combined in a large glass jar: add the ginger pieces, starting tea, filtered water, and sweet tea.
- Add SCOBY: Lightly lay the SCOBY over the mixture. To prevent contamination, always wash your hands and your utensils.

- Cover and Ferment: Place a cloth or paper towel over the jar and fasten it with a string or rubber band. Depending on the degree of fermentation you want, leave the jar in a warm, dark place for seven to fourteen days.

- Taste Test: After the initial fermentation, taste the kombucha. If it's to your liking, remove the SCOBY. If not, let it ferment longer.

- Bottle and Carbonate: Transfer the kombucha to smaller glass bottles, leaving about an inch of space at the top. Optionally, add flavorings like more ginger or fruits. Seal the bottles tightly and let them carbonate for 2-7 days.

- Refrigerate: Once carbonated, refrigerate the bottles to slow down fermentation and chill the kombucha.

Time of Preparation:

- Approximately 1-2 weeks, depending on your desired fermentation level.

Tips and Tricks:

- Use clean utensils and jars to prevent contamination.

- Experiment with ginger quantity for personalized flavor.

- Maintain a consistent brewing temperature for best results.

Nutritional Value (Per Serving):

- Calories: ~30

- Sugar: ~5g

- Probiotics: Varies based on fermentation duration

Health Benefits:

- Rich in probiotics for gut health.

- Antioxidants from tea and ginger.

- Potential anti-inflammatory properties.

Packaging and Storing:

- Store in airtight glass bottles to maintain carbonation.

- Refrigerate to extend shelf life.

- Keep away from direct sunlight.

Precautions:

- Ensure cleanliness to prevent contamination.

- If unsure, consult a healthcare professional before consuming.

Post-Caution:

- Start with small amounts to gauge tolerance.

- Discontinue if adverse reactions occur.

- Eat in moderation as part of a well-rounded diet.

Homemade Coconut Milk Kefir

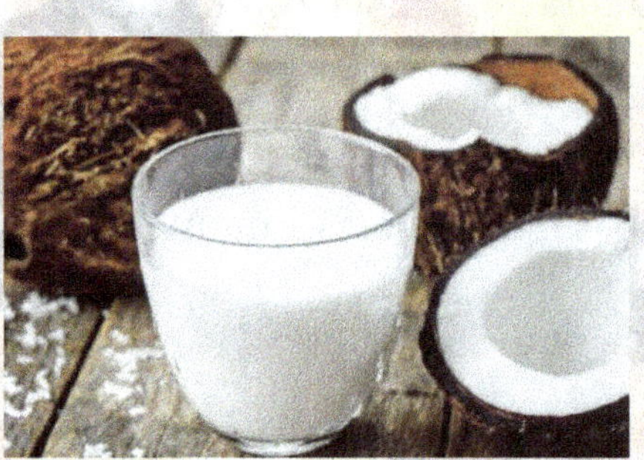

Ingredients:

- 2 cups of unsweetened coconut milk

- 1-2 tablespoons of kefir grains

- 1 teaspoon of sugar (for the fermentation process)

- Glass jar with a lid

- Wooden or plastic stirring utensil

- Cheesecloth or coffee filter

- Rubber band or string

- Prepare Coconut Milk: Ensure the coconut milk is unsweetened. If it's canned, shake well before using. If using homemade coconut milk, ensure it's at room temperature.

- Add Kefir Grains: Place the kefir grains into the glass jar.

- Combine Ingredients: Pour the coconut milk into the jar, add the sugar, and stir gently with a wooden or plastic utensil. Avoid metal utensils as they can damage kefir grains.

- Cover and Ferment: Tighten the jar with a rubber band or string after covering it with two layers of cheesecloth or a coffee filter. Depending on the degree of fermentation you want, let it ferment for 12 to 48 hours at room temperature.

- Strain Kefir Grains: After fermentation, strain the kefir grains from the liquid using a plastic or wooden sieve.

- Bottle and Refrigerate: Transfer the liquid into a sealed glass bottle and refrigerate. This slows down the fermentation process.

Time of Preparation:

- Approximately 1-2 days, including fermentation time.

Tips and Tricks:

- Use quality kefir grains for optimal fermentation.

- Experiment with fermentation time for varied consistency and flavor.
- Store kefir grains in a separate container with fresh coconut milk for future use.

Nutritional Value (Per Serving):

- Calories: ~50
- Healthy fats: ~5g
- Probiotics: Abundant, aiding in digestion and gut health.

Health Benefits:

- Promotes gut health with live probiotics.
- Potential immune system support.
- Rich in vitamins and minerals from coconut milk.

Packaging and Storing:

- Use a sealed glass bottle for storing in the refrigerator.
- Shake well before consuming to mix any separated layers.
- Consume within 1-2 weeks for optimal freshness.

Precautions:

- Ensure the cleanliness of utensils and jar to prevent contamination.
- Monitor fermentation time to avoid over-fermentation.

Post-Caution:

- Start with small amounts to gauge tolerance.
- If new to kefir, introduce gradually to your diet.
- Consult a healthcare professional if you have concerns about dairy substitutes.

Berry Probiotic Smoothie

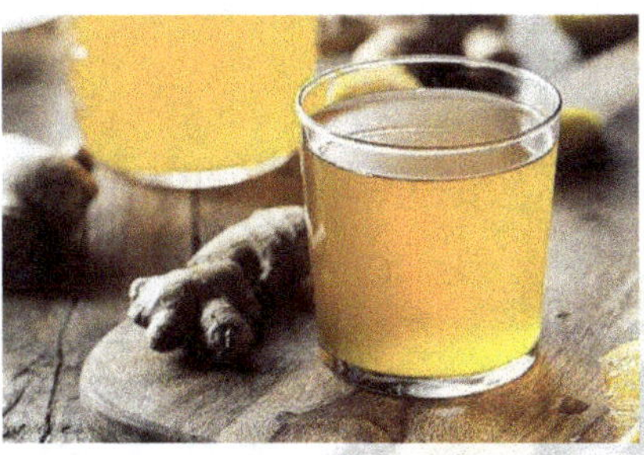

Ingredients:

- 1 cup mixed berries (strawberries, blueberries, raspberries)
- 1 ripe banana
- 1 cup plain yogurt or kefir
- 1 tablespoon chia seeds
- 1 tablespoon honey (optional, for sweetness)
- Half a cup almond milk, or any other preferred beverage
- Ice cubes (optional)

Procedure:

- Prepare Ingredients: Wash and hull the berries. Peel and slice the banana.
- Blend Ingredients: In a blender, combine the mixed berries, banana, yogurt or kefir, chia seeds, honey (if using), and almond milk. Blend until smooth.
- Modify Texture: In case the smoothie is excessively thick, incorporate extra liquid, or if it's too thin, add more fruit. Repeat blending until the desired consistency is reached.
- Add Ice Cubes (Optional): For a colder and thicker smoothie, add ice cubes and blend until smooth.

- Serve Immediately: Pour the smoothie into a glass and enjoy immediately.

Time of Preparation:

- Approximately 5-10 minutes.

Tips and Tricks:

- Use frozen berries for a colder and thicker smoothie.
- Experiment with different berries for varied flavors.
- Adjust sweetness with honey according to personal preference.

Nutritional Value (Per Serving):

- Calories: ~200
- Fiber: ~6g
- Probiotics: Abundant, contributing to gut health.
- Vitamins and Antioxidants: From berries, promoting overall well-being.

Health Benefits:

- Provides a rich source of antioxidants.
- Supports digestive health with probiotics.
- Nutrient-dense with vitamins and minerals.

Packaging and Storing:

- Best consumed immediately for freshness.
- If preparing in advance, store in an airtight container in the refrigerator for up to 24 hours.
- Shake or stir before consuming if any separation occurs.

Precautions:

- Be cautious with added sweeteners if watching sugar intake.

- Check for allergies or sensitivities to specific berries.

Post-Caution:

- Enjoy as part of a balanced diet.
- Monitor portion sizes if considering calorie intake.
- Should any unfavorable responses arise, seek advice from a medical expert.

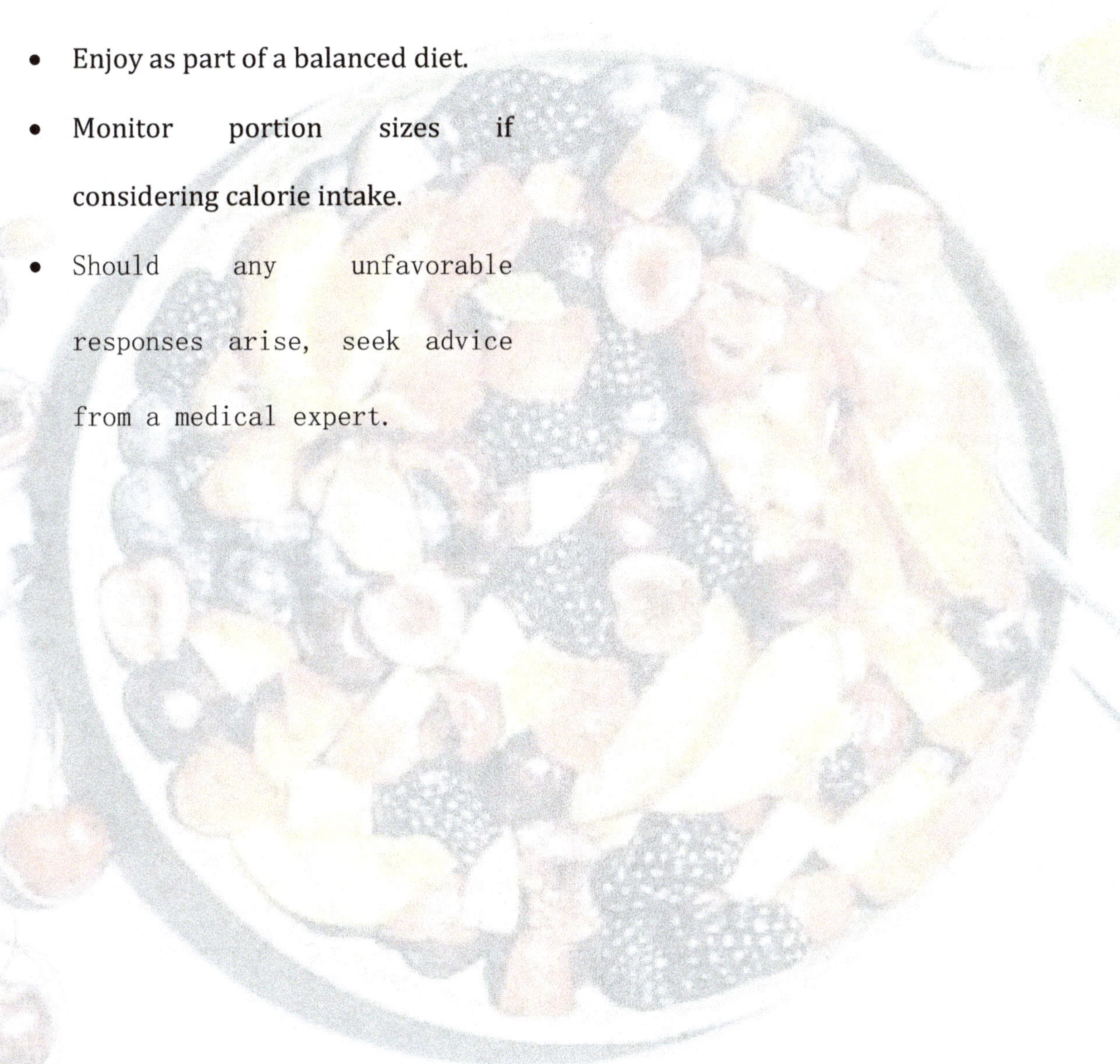

7

GAPS Desserts

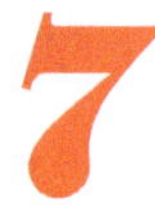

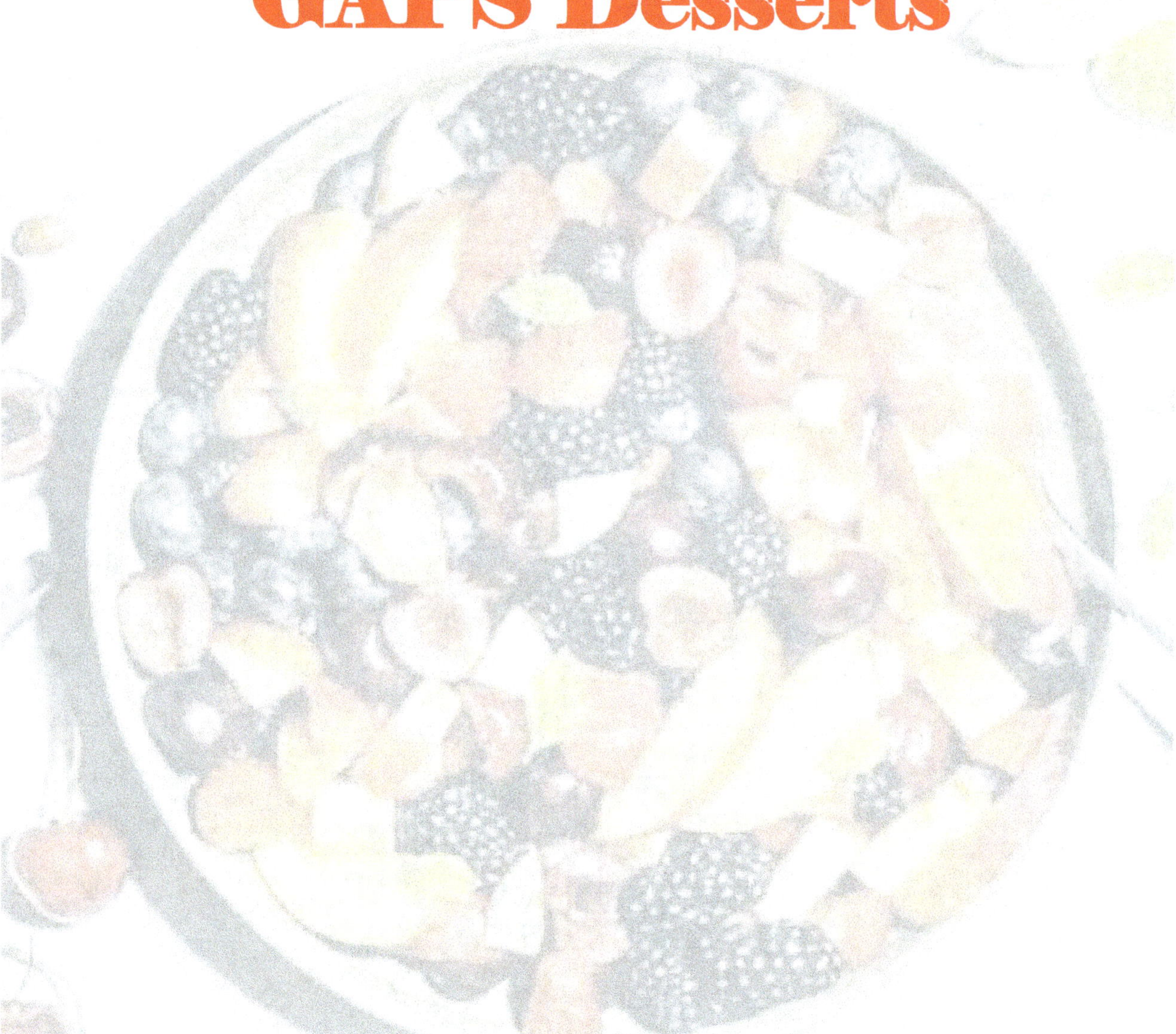

Gut-Healing Apple Crisp

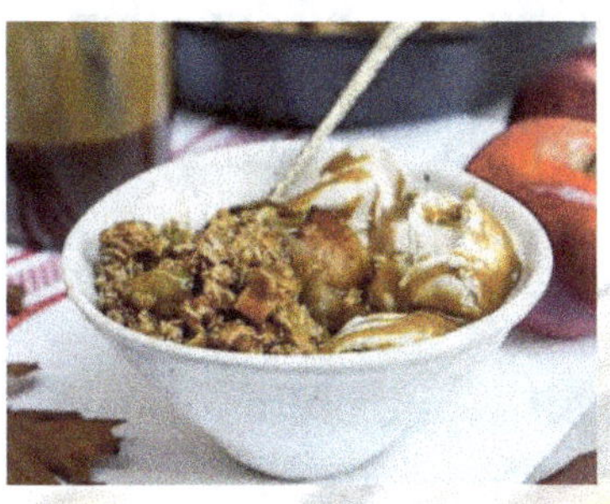

Ingredients:

- 6 medium-sized apples, peeled, cored, and sliced
- 1 cup almond flour
- 1 cup rolled oats
- 1/2 cup coconut sugar
- 1/2 cup melted coconut oil
- 1 teaspoon ground cinnamon
- 1/2 teaspoon ground ginger
- 1/4 teaspoon sea salt
- 1/2 cup chopped walnuts (optional)

Procedure:

- Preheat the oven to 350°F (175°C).

- Combine sliced apples, ginger, and cinnamon in a large bowl. Place them in a baking dish, evenly spaced.

- In another bowl, mix almond flour, rolled oats, coconut sugar, melted coconut oil, and sea salt until a crumbly texture is formed.

- Sprinkle the oat mixture over the apples, ensuring an even layer.

- Optional: Add chopped walnuts for an extra crunch.

- Bake for 40-45 minutes or until the topping is golden brown and the apples are tender.

- Before serving, let it cool for a few minutes.

Time of Preparation:

- Approximately 20 minutes for preparation, 40-45 minutes for baking.

Tips and Tricks:

- Choose apples rich in fiber, like Granny Smith or Pink Lady, for added gut health benefits.
- Adjust sweetness by altering the amount of coconut sugar according to taste preference.
- Experiment with different nuts for varied textures.

Nutritional Value (Per Serving):

- Calories: 280
- Protein: 4g
- Fat: 15g
- Carbohydrates: 35g
- Fiber: 6g

Health Benefits:

- Almond flour provides a gluten-free alternative, aiding digestion.
- Oats contain beta-glucans, promoting gut health.
- Coconut oil contributes healthy fats with antimicrobial properties.

Packaging and Storing:

- Allow the crisp to cool completely before storing in an airtight container.
- For extended shelf life, freeze or refrigerate for up to three days. **Precautions:**
- Individuals with nut allergies should opt for alternative flours.
- Monitor sugar intake if following a low-sugar diet.

Post-Caution:

- Listen to your body's response; if any discomfort occurs, consult a healthcare professional.

- Share and enjoy this gut-healing apple crisp responsibly.

Avocado Chocolate Mousse

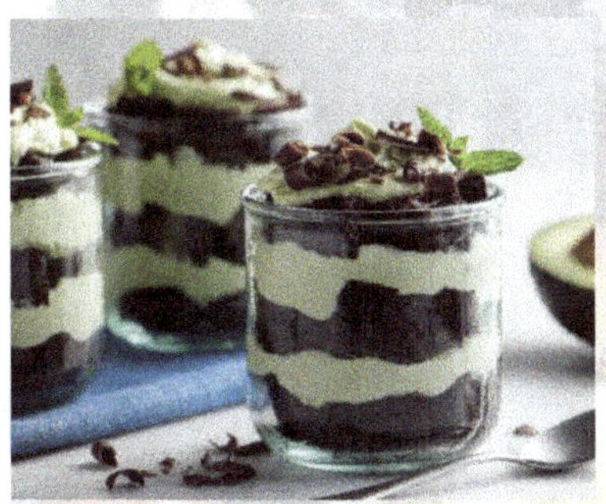

Ingredients:

- 2 ripe avocados, peeled and pitted

- 1/2 cup unsweetened cocoa powder

- 1/2 cup maple syrup or agave nectar

- 1/4 cup almond milk

- 1 teaspoon vanilla extract

- A pinch of sea salt

- Optional toppings: berries, chopped nuts, or coconut flakes

Procedure:

- In a blender or food processor, combine avocados, cocoa powder, maple syrup, almond milk, vanilla extract, and sea salt. Scrape down the sides as necessary, then blend until smooth and creamy.

If necessary, adjust the sweetness or consistency by adding additional sweetener or almond milk.

Transfer the mousse into bowls

or serving glasses, and then chill it for a minimum of two hours to allow it to solidify. Before serving, garnish with coconut flakes, chopped almonds, or berries.

Time of Preparation:

- Approximately 10 minutes for preparation, 2 hours for chilling.

Tips and Tricks:

- Ensure avocados are fully ripe for a smoother texture.
- Experiment with different sweeteners based on your preference.
- Adjust cocoa powder quantity for desired chocolate intensity.

Nutritional Value (Per Serving):

- Calories: 200
- Protein: 3g
- Fat: 15g
- Carbohydrates: 20g
- Fiber: 7g

Health Benefits:

- Avocados provide healthy monounsaturated fats and fiber.
- Cocoa powder is rich in antioxidants and may have cardiovascular benefits.
- Low in added sugars compared to traditional chocolate desserts.

Packaging and Storing:

- Keep refrigerated in sealed containers for a maximum of 48 hours.
- Note: Avocado-based desserts may oxidize, so consume promptly for optimal freshness.

Precautions:

- Monitor portion sizes, especially for individuals on calorie-restricted diets.

- Check for allergies to any ingredients, especially avocados.

Post-Caution:

- Enjoy this guilt-free indulgence but be mindful of overall dietary balance.

- Should any unfavorable responses arise, seek advice from a medical expert. **This**

Coconut Flour Blueberry Muffins

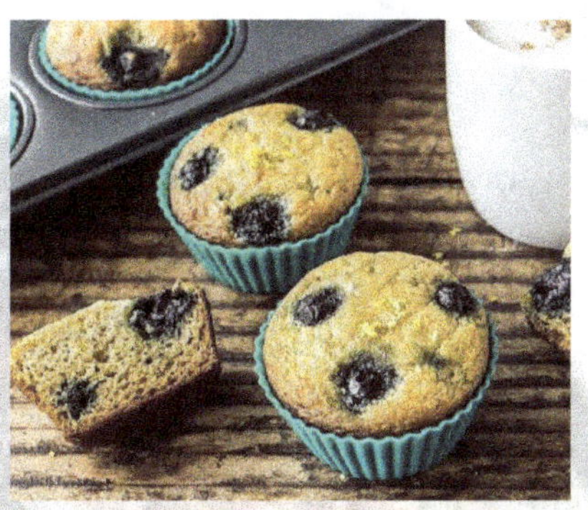

Ingredients:

- 1/2 cup coconut flour

- 1/4 cup almond flour

- 1/2 teaspoon baking soda

- 1/4 teaspoon salt

- 4 large eggs

- 1/4 cup coconut oil, melted

- 1/3 cup maple syrup or honey

- 1 teaspoon vanilla extract

- 1 cup fresh or frozen blueberries

Procedure:

- Preheat the oven to 350°F (175°C) and line a muffin tin with paper liners.

- In a bowl, whisk together coconut flour, almond flour, baking soda, and salt.

- In a separate bowl, whisk eggs, melted coconut oil, maple syrup (or honey), and vanilla extract until well combined.

- Blend the dry components with the wet ones until a smooth consistency is achieved. Fold in the blueberries gently. Evenly distribute the batter among the muffin cups. Preheat the oven to 200 – 250 degrees Fahrenheit, or until a toothpick inserted in the center emerges clean.

Before moving the muffins to a wire rack, let them cool in the muffin tray for five minutes.

Time of Preparation:

- Approximately 15 minutes for preparation, 20-25 minutes for baking.

Tips and Tricks:

- Coconut flour absorbs moisture, so be cautious not to overmix the batter.

- Adjust sweetness by varying the amount of maple syrup or honey.

- For added texture, sprinkle shredded coconut on top before baking.

Nutritional Value (Per Serving):

- Calories: 120

- Protein: 4g

- Fat: 8g

- Carbohydrates: 10g

- Fiber: 3g

Health Benefits:

- Coconut flour is a good source of fiber and lower in carbohydrates.

- Almond flour provides healthy fats and adds a nutty flavor.

- Blueberries are rich in antioxidants and vitamins.

Packaging and Storing:

- Store in an airtight container at room temperature for up to 3 days, or refrigerate for longer freshness.

Precautions:

- Ensure coconut flour is well sifted to avoid lumps.

- Check for allergies, especially for individuals sensitive to nuts or eggs.

Post-Caution:

- Enjoy these Coconut Flour Blueberry Muffins as a nutritious snack or breakfast option.

- Should any unfavorable responses arise, seek advice from a medical expert.

8

Special Occasion Treats

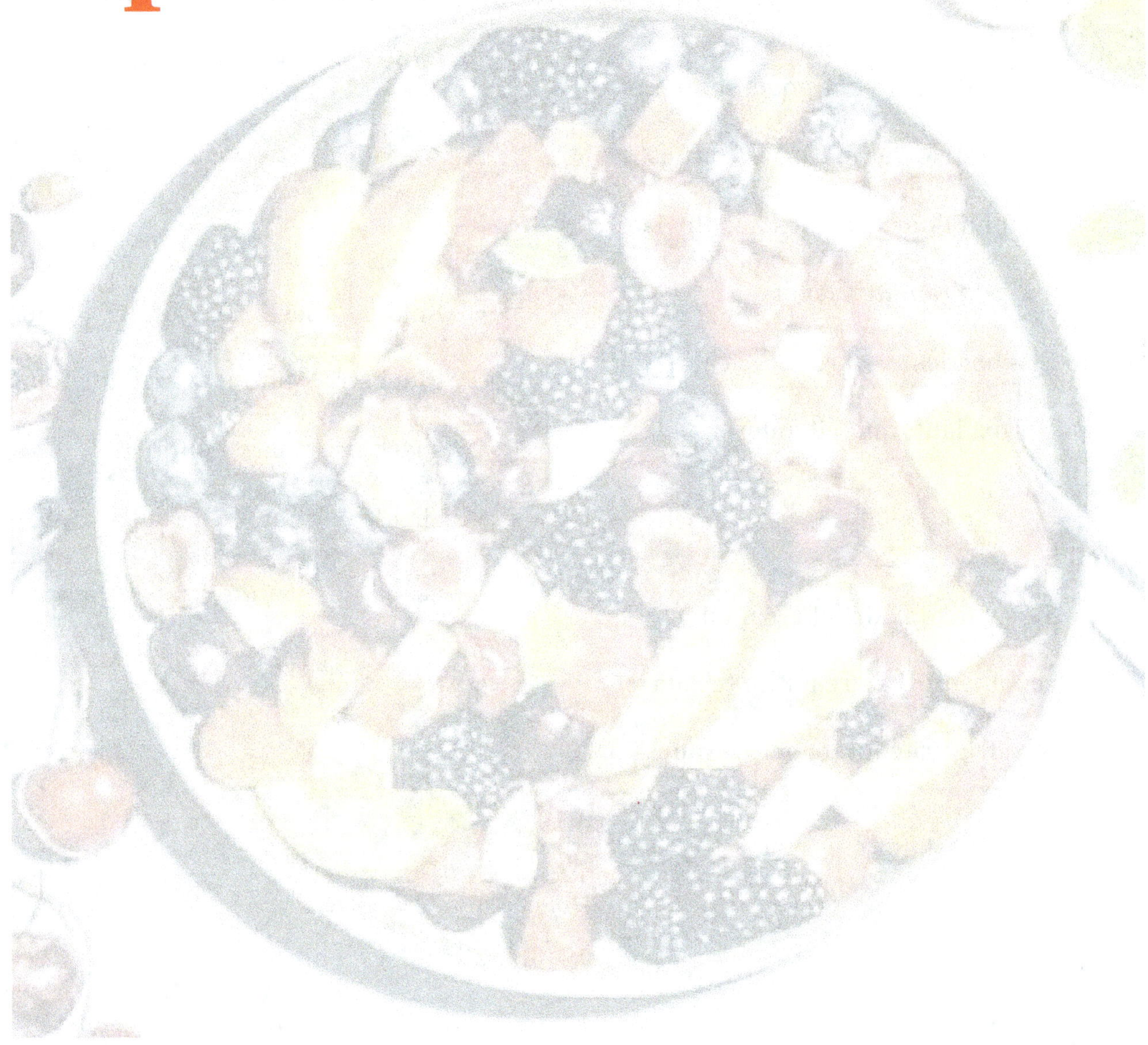

Gut-Friendly Pumpkin Pie

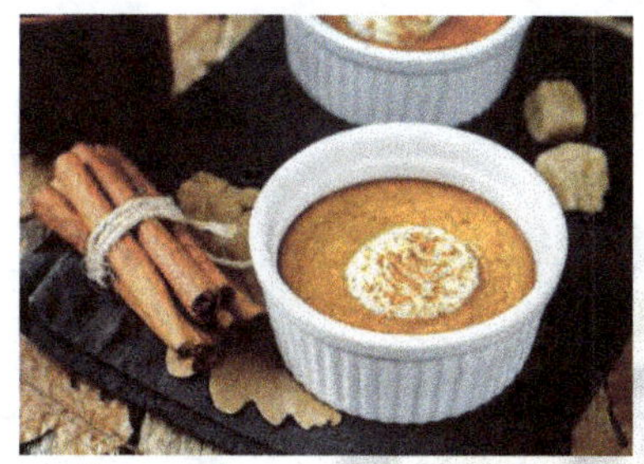

Ingredients:

- 2 cups canned pumpkin puree
- 3/4 cup coconut milk (or any non-dairy milk)
- 1/2 cup pure maple syrup
- 1/4 cup coconut flour
- 2 teaspoons pumpkin pie spice
- 1 teaspoon vanilla extract
- 1/2 teaspoon sea salt
- 3 eggs
- 1 gluten-free pie crust

Procedure:

- Set the oven temperature to 350° F (175° C).

Pumpkin puree, coconut milk, maple syrup, coconut flour, pumpkin pie spice, vanilla essence, and sea salt should all be combined in a big basin. One egg at a time, adding and thoroughly mixing after each addition.

Transfer the blend into the ready-made gluten-free pie shell.

Bake for forty-five to fifty minutes, or until the middle sets.

Let the pie cool completely before cutting.

Time of Preparation:

- Approximately 1 hour (including baking time).

Tips and Tricks:

- Use a high-quality gluten-free pie crust for the best results.

- Adjust sweetness by adding more or less maple syrup based on your preference.

- For a smoother texture, blend the pumpkin mixture in a food processor before pouring into the pie crust.

Nutritional Value per Serving:

- Calories: 220

- Protein: 4g

- Fat: 12g

- Carbohydrates: 25g

- Fiber: 3g

- Sugars: 15g

Health Benefits:

- Rich in beta-carotene from pumpkin, promoting eye health.

- Coconut flour provides fiber, supporting gut health.

- Maple syrup offers antioxidants and minerals.

Packaging and Storing:

- Store the pumpkin pie in an airtight container in the refrigerator for up to 3 days.

- For longer storage, freeze individual slices, wrapped in plastic and aluminum foil.

Precautions:

- Ensure all ingredients are gluten-free if following a gluten-free diet.

- Check the consistency of the pie filling; it should be firm but not overbaked.

Post-Caution:

- If experiencing digestive discomfort, monitor ingredients

and portion sizes to identify potential triggers.

- In the event that stomach problems persist, get medical advice.

Almond Flour Birthday Cake

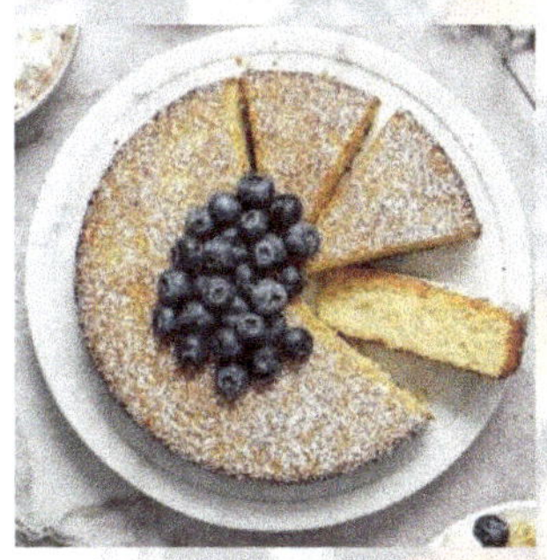

Ingredients:

- 2 1/2 cups almond flour
- 1/2 cup coconut flour
- 1 teaspoon baking powder
- 1/2 teaspoon baking soda
- 1/2 teaspoon salt
- 1/2 cup unsalted butter, softened
- 1 cup granulated sweetener (e.g., erythritol or monk fruit)
- 4 large eggs
- 1 cup unsweetened almond milk
- 1 teaspoon vanilla extract

Procedure:

- Set the oven temperature to 350° F (175° C). Grease two 8-inch cake pans, and line them. Mix the almond flour, coconut flour, baking soda, baking powder, and salt in a bowl. Beat the softened butter and sweetener together in a large, separate dish until they become light and fluffy. Beat thoroughly after adding each egg one at a time. Add the dry ingredients to the wet ingredients gradually, mixing in almond milk in between each addition. With the dry ingredients, start and finish.

Add vanilla extract and stir.

Evenly divide the batter among the cake pans that have been prepared.

When a toothpick put into the center comes out clean, bake for 25 to 30 minutes.

Before icing, let the cakes cool fully.

Time preparation

- is around one hour, which includes the baking and cooling periods.).

Tips and Tricks:

- Use room temperature ingredients for better incorporation.
- Add a touch of lemon zest for a citrusy flavor.
- Frost the cake with a cream cheese or almond butter frosting for extra richness.

Nutritional Value per Serving:

- Calories: 280
- Protein: 8g
- Fat: 24g
- Carbohydrates: 10g
- Fiber: 4g
- Sugars: 1g

Health Benefits:

- Almond flour is an excellent source of protein and beneficial lipids.

- Low in carbohydrates, suitable for those following a low-carb or keto lifestyle.

- Enjoy in moderation, and consult a healthcare professional if following a specific dietary plan.

Packaging and Storing:

- Store the almond flour birthday cake in an airtight container in the refrigerator for up to 5 days.

- Freeze individual slices for longer storage, wrapped in plastic and aluminum foil.

Precautions:

- Ensure all ingredients are fresh, especially the almond flour.

- Adjust sweetener quantity based on personal taste preferences.

Post-Caution:

- Monitor sugar intake, especially if using sweeteners, to avoid excessive consumption.

Celebratory Fruit Salad

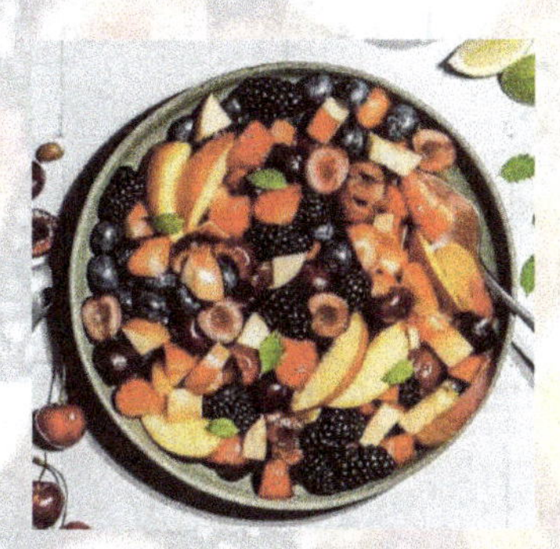

Ingredients:

- 2 cups strawberries, hulled and halved

- 1 cup blueberries

- 1 cup green grapes, halved

- 1 cup pineapple chunks

- 1 cup kiwi, peeled and sliced

- 1 cup mango, peeled and diced

- 1 tablespoon honey or maple syrup (optional)
- Fresh mint leaves for garnish

Procedure:

- Wash and prepare all the fruits as instructed.
- In a large bowl, gently combine strawberries, blueberries, green grapes, pineapple, kiwi, and mango.
- If desired, drizzle honey or maple syrup over the fruit and gently toss to coat.
- For a taste explosion, add some fresh mint leaves as a garnish. Refrigerate for at least 30 minutes before serving to enhance flavors.

Time of Preparation:

- Approximately 15-20 minutes (excluding refrigeration time).

Tips and Tricks:

- Choose ripe and colorful fruits for the best taste and presentation.
- Experiment with different fruit combinations based on seasonal availability.
- For a zesty touch, pour in some fresh lime juice.

Nutritional Value per Serving:

- Calories: 120
- Protein: 2g
- Fat: 0.5g
- Carbohydrates: 30g
- Fiber: 4g
- Sugars: 22g

Health Benefits:

- Rich in vitamins, minerals, and antioxidants from a variety of fruits.
- High fiber content supports digestive health.

- Natural sugars provide a healthier alternative to processed desserts.

Packaging and Storing:

- Serve the celebratory fruit salad in a decorative bowl or individual cups for an appealing presentation.
- Store any leftovers in the refrigerator for up to two days in an airtight container.

Precautions:

- Check for allergies among guests and customize the fruit selection accordingly.
- Avoid overripe fruits to maintain freshness.

Post-Caution:

- Monitor portion sizes, especially for those managing blood sugar levels.

- Enjoy the fruit salad as part of a balanced diet.
- Celebrate joyous occasions with this vibrant and refreshing celebratory fruit salad!

4 weeks meal plan

Week 1:

Day 1:

- Breakfast: Homemade Yogurt with Berry Probiotic Smoothie

- Lunch: Quinoa and Roasted Veggie Bowl

- Dinner: Baked Salmon with Lemon and Herbs

Day 2:

- Breakfast: Gut-Supporting Energy Bites

- Lunch: Lentil and Spinach Stew

- Dinner: Grass-Fed Beef Stir-Fry with Vegetables

Day 3:

- Breakfast: Avocado Chocolate Mousse

- Lunch: Butternut Squash & Carrot Immunity Soup

- Dinner: Sauerkraut with Probiotic Goodness

Day 4:

- Breakfast: Coconut Flour Blueberry Muffins

- Lunch: Cauliflower Rice Pilaf for Gut Health

- Dinner: Turkey and Sweet Potato Casserole

Week 2:

Day 5:

- Breakfast: Gut-Healing Apple Crisp

- Lunch: Homemade Coconut Milk Kefir

- Dinner: Creamy Zucchini Soup for Gut Nourishment

Day 6:

- Breakfast: Berry Probiotic Smoothie

- Lunch: Almond Flour Crackers with Avocado and Salsa Dip

- Dinner: Grass-Fed Beef Stir-Fry with Vegetables

Day 7:

- Breakfast: Ginger Kombucha Elixir

- Lunch: Lentil and Spinach Stew

- Dinner: Baked Salmon with Lemon and Herbs

Day 8:

- Breakfast: Almond Flour Birthday Cake

- Lunch: Quinoa and Roasted Veggie Bowl

- Dinner: Butternut Squash & Carrot Immunity Soup

Week 3:

Day 9:

- Breakfast: Homemade Yogurt with Berry Probiotic Smoothie

- Lunch: Avocado and Salsa Dip with Fermented Pickles

- Dinner: Gut Healing Chicken Soup

Day 10:

- Breakfast: Coconut Flour Blueberry Muffins

- Lunch: Cauliflower Rice Pilaf for Gut Health

- Dinner: Turkey and Sweet Potato Casserole

Day 11:

- Breakfast: Gut-Supporting Energy Bites

- Lunch: Lentil and Spinach Stew

- Dinner: Creamy Zucchini Soup for Gut Nourishment

Day 12:

- Breakfast: Avocado Chocolate Mousse

- Lunch: Quinoa and Roasted Veggie Bowl

- Dinner: Baked Salmon with Lemon and Herbs

Week 4:

Day 13:

- Breakfast: Berry Probiotic Smoothie

- Lunch: Almond Flour Crackers with Avocado and Salsa Dip

- Dinner: Grass-Fed Beef Stir-Fry with Vegetables

Day 14:

- Breakfast: Ginger Kombucha Elixir

- Lunch: Butternut Squash & Carrot Immunity Soup

- Dinner: Sauerkraut with Probiotic Goodness

Day 15:

- Breakfast: Almond Flour Birthday Cake

- Lunch: Homemade Coconut Milk Kefir

- Dinner: Gut Healing Chicken Soup

Day 16:

- Breakfast: Gut-Healing Apple Crisp

- Lunch: Fermented Pickles with Cauliflower Rice Pilaf for Gut Health

- Dinner: Turkey and Sweet Potato Casserole

CONCLUSION

The GAPS cookbook serves as a valuable resource for enhancing gut health through nourishing and flavorful recipes. With its carefully crafted collection of dishes, designed to support the gut-brain connection, this cookbook not only provides a culinary journey but also empowers individuals to prioritize their well-being. By embracing the principles of the Gut and Psychology Syndrome (GAPS) diet, readers can embark on a delicious path towards improved digestive health, fostering a holistic approach to wellness. The diverse and appealing recipes within this cookbook not only cater to nutritional needs but also make the journey towards gut health an enjoyable and satisfying experience.

www.ingramcontent.com/pod-product-compliance
Lightning Source LLC
Chambersburg PA
CBHW080725260726
48660CB00010B/3696